The Paleo Ketogenic Holiday Recipes for Beginners

IMPORTANT INFORMATION

The information provided in this book is designed to provide helpful information on the subjects discussed. This book is not meant to be used, nor should it be used, to diagnose or treat any medical condition. For diagnosis or treatment of any medical problem, consult your own physician. The publisher and author are not responsible for any specific health or allergy needs that may require medical supervision and are not liable for any damages or negative consequences from any treatment, action, application or preparation, to any person reading or following the information in this book. References are provided for informational purposes only and do not constitute endorsement of any websites or other sources. Readers should be aware that the websites listed in this book may change.

FREE GIFT

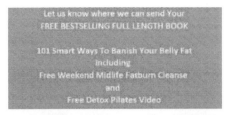

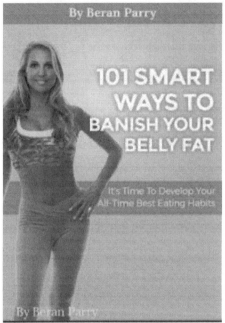

Please search this page over the internet
forms.aweber.com/form/14/395417614.htm

The Paleo Ketogenic Holiday Recipes for Beginners By Beran Parry

WHAT THIS BOOK IS NOT!

Whilst I have referred where appropriate to important medically based studies, books and medical papers, this book has not been written as a medical research paper, designed to cover dozens of scientific subjects.

I have deliberately avoided the current trend in many diet books to constantly cherry pick medical and scientific studies to support the book's conclusions. This book is not intended as a reference item to satisfy those readers that might be looking for useful research material.

There will be a detailed bibliography attached to this book. This is a truly exciting and rapidly evolving science and there is a vast amount of material to read and study about Epigenetics and Functional Medicine in general, especially in the way that these insights apply to intelligent weight management. If you require further information, I suggest you contact me for specific recommendations at beranparry@gmail.com

The Paleo Ketogenic Holiday Recipes for Beginners By Beran Parry

Copyright © 2017 by Beran Parry

(olw112017)

All rights reserved. No part of this publication may be reproduced, distributed, or transmitted in any form or by any means, including photocopying, recording, or other electronic or mechanical methods, without the prior written permission of the publisher, except in the case of brief quotations embodied in critical reviews and certain other non-commercial uses permitted by copyright law. For permission requests, write to the author's email address: beranparry@gmail.com

The Paleo Ketogenic Holiday Recipes for Beginners By Beran Parry

FOR MORE FROM BERAN PARRY

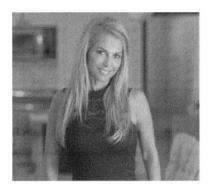

Please search this page over the www.amazon.com

beranparry.com/

The Paleo Ketogenic Holiday Recipes for Beginners By Beran Parry

The Paleo Ketogenic Holiday Recipes for Beginners

By

Beran Parry

The Paleo Ketogenic Holiday Recipes for Beginners By Beran Parry

Foreword

One of the most frequent objections I hear about the Paleo Diet is that the ingredients cost too much. There's a definite perception out there that the Paleo Diet is somehow too expensive and unaffordable. But what if that simply isn't true? What if it's possible to enjoy all the incredible benefits of smart nutrition and stay easily within your usual food budget range? Not only is it possible, it's highly desirable and I'm going to show you how.

The recipes in this fabulous book will also show you how to enjoy mealtimes to the max and still fuel your body with the best nutrition it can get. This is how to celebrate Thanksgiving and Xmas in style! Celebrate with great food and totally natural weight loss. Enjoy every single mouthful from this stellar collection of super-nutritious recipes and feel energised as your body burns off the excess fat. Celebrate your return to the smartest way to feed your body. Make Thanksgiving a day to remember as you celebrate the gift of your health and a naturally leaner, trimmer, healthier body. And that's something you can celebrate every single day;

Our bodies haven't changed much since those ancient days so we know how tough it is on our digestive systems to feed ourselves with sugars and carbs and processed food that upsets the balance of our digestive systems and leads to inflammation throughout our bodies. Sounds serious but it's such an easy problem to solve. Our bodies developed and prospered on a diet that was free from processed foods, that was low on carbs, that rarely contained any kind of sugar or dairy products. We thrived on a diet of protein and fat and ate lots of plants and vegetables.

Thanksgiving and Xmas are just around the corner and it's time to break out the party hats and celebrate this important day with truly delicious food that will boost your health and still melt away the excess pounds. Wait a second. Did you just say `delicious food` and `melt away the excess pounds`? At the same time? Is that really possible? Oh, yes it is! That's exactly right. Now you can enjoy the most wonderful meals and still burn off the weight, say goodbye to your old belly fat, boost your health, have a great time and feel amazing. And how do we do that? Easy. All you need is the new **Paleo Ketogenic Holiday Recipes for Beginners**. You see, your body knows exactly what it needs to be strong and lean and healthy.

The Paleo Ketogenic Holiday Recipes for Beginners By Beran Parry

Table of Contents

Foreword 8
AcknowledgementS FOR MY PALEO AND RECIPE RESEARCH 14
Preface 15
CHAPTER 1 17
   About Beran 17
Chapter 2 23
   So Why Can't I Lose Weight? And why can't I keep the weight off? 23
Chapter 3 27
   Epigenetics + Long Term Eating Behaviours = Your Present Weight Level 27
Chapter 4 29
   You are now Managing Director of Your Paleo Delicious Life. Inc. 29
   The Paleo Delicious Epigenetic Shopping Guide 29
Chapter 5 – 31
   Paleo Budget Tips 31
Chapter 6 – 33
   RECIPES 33
   Holiday Breakfasts (Grain Free) 33
     1. Apple Celebration Dream 33
     2. Party Protein Muesli 34
     3. Celebratory Apple Almond Coconut Medley 35
   Holiday Egg Meals 36
     4. Latina Eggs with Chilli 36
     5. Basil and Walnut Eggs Divine 37
     6. Spicy Sumptious Eggs 38
     7. Spicy India Egg Party 39
     8. Spectacular Spinach Omelet 40
     9. Blushing Blueberry Omelet 41
     10. Holiday Supercharger Omelet with Fennel and Dill 42
     11. Outstanding Veggie Omelet 43
     12. Spicy Spinach Bake 44

The Paleo Ketogenic Holiday Recipes for Beginners By Beran Parry

13.	Post Thanksgiving Veggie Hash With Eggs	45
14.	Spectacular Eggie Salsa	46
15.	Mushrooms, Eggs and Onion Bonanza	47
16.	Celebratory Avocado and Shrimp Omelet	48
17.	Delish Veggie Breakfast Peppers	49
18.	Breakfast Mexicana Fiesta	50
19.	Zucchini Party Casserole	51
20.	Blueberry Nut Casserole	52

Holiday Main Course (Lunch or Dinner) 53

Turkey and Chicken Meals 53

21.	Spicy Holiday Turkey Stir Fry	53
22.	Party Roasted Lemon Herb Chicken	54
23.	Roasted and Filled Bell Peppers Feast	55
24.	Party Pasta and Turkey Bolognaise	56
25.	Thanksgiving Turkey Spaghetti Squash Boats	57
26.	Tantalizing Turkey Party Stir-fry	58
27.	Sexy Turkey Scramble	59
28.	Chicken Fennel Feast	60

Holiday Starter Course - Fish 61

29.	Tempting Thai Baked Fish with Squash Noodles	61
30.	Superior Salmon with Lemon and Thyme OR Use any White fish	63
31.	Party Delish Baked dill Salmon	64
32.	Holiday Salmon in Herb Crust	65
33.	Salmon Mustard Delish	66
34.	Garlic Lemon Shrimp Bonanza	67
35.	Celebratory Courgette Pesto and Shrimp	68
36.	Cheeky Curry Shrimp	69
37.	Sexy Shrimp on Sticks	70

Holiday Starter Salad – Animal Protein 71

38.	Delicious Slaw	71
39.	Tastylicious Cabbage Salad	72

The Paleo Ketogenic Holiday Recipes for Beginners By Beran Parry

40.	Chicken Basil Avo Salad	73
41.	Thanksgiving Turkey Taco Salad	74
42.	Macadamia Chicken Salad	75
43.	Turkey Sprouts Salad	76
44.	Avocado Tuna Salad	77
45.	Asian Aspiration Salad	78
46.	Creamy Carrot Salad	79
47.	Tasty Tuna Stuffed Tomato	80

Holiday Desserts 81

48.	Rose Banana Delicious Brownies	81
49.	Secret Sumptious Brownies	82
50.	Choco-coco Brownies	83
51.	Coco – Walnut Brownie Bites	84
52.	Party Peach and Almond Cake	85
53.	Fetching Fudge	86
54.	Choco – Almond Delights	87
55.	Peachy Creamy Peaches	88
56.	Lemon-Coconut Petit Fours	89

Holiday Snacks 91

57.	Holiday Breakfast Bonanza Muffins	91
58.	Perfect Pumpkin Seeds	92
59.	Gorgeous Spicy Nuts	93
60.	Krunchy Yummy Kale Chips	94
61.	Divine Butternut Chips	95
62.	Outstanding Orange Snack	96
63.	Pumpkin Vanilla Delight	97
64.	Delectable Parsnip Chips	98
65.	Anti-Aging Fruit Delights	99
66.	Power Snack	100
67.	Delish Cashew Butter Treats	101

Holiday Smoothie Delight 102

The Paleo Ketogenic Holiday Recipes for Beginners By Beran Parry

68. Gorgeous Berry Smoothie 102
69. Tempting Coconut Berry Smoothie 103
70. Volumptious Vanilla Hot Drink 104
71. Almond Butter Smoothies 105
72. Choco Walnut Delight 106
73. Raspberry Hemp Smoothie 107
74. Choco Banana Smoothie 108
75. Blueberry Almond Smoothie 109
76. Hazelnut Butter and Banana Smoothie 110
77. Vanilla Blueberry Smoothie 111
78. Chocolate Raspberry Smoothie 112
79. Peach Smoothie 113
80. Zesty Citrus Smoothie 114
81. Apple Smoothie 115
82. Pineapple Smoothie 116
83. Strawberry Smoothie 117
84. Pineapple Coconut Deluxe Smoothie 118
85. Divine Vanilla Smoothie 119
86. Coco Orange Delish Smoothie 120
87. Baby Kale Pineapple Smoothie 121
88. Sumptuous Strawberry Coconut Smoothie 122
89. Blueberry Bonanza Smoothies 123
90. Divine Peach Coconut Smoothie 124
91. Tantalizing Key Lime Pie Smoothie 125
92. High Protein and Nutritional Delish Smoothie 126
93. Pineapple Protein Smoothie 127
94. Raspberry Coconut Smoothie 128
95. Ginger Carrot Protein Smoothie 129

Holiday Sumptuous Soup 130

96. Wonderful Watercress Soup 130
97. Celery Cashew Cream Soup 131

98.	Tempting Tomato Basil Soup	132
99.	Delicious Lemon-Garlic Soup	133
100.	Turkey Squash Soup	134

Bibliography 135

BEFORE YOU GO 136

The Paleo Ketogenic Holiday Recipes for Beginners By Beran Parry

AcknowledgementS FOR MY PALEO AND RECIPE RESEARCH

The inspiration to write this book began more than thirty years ago when I embarked on my first nutritional science courses under the tutelage of Dr Boris Chaitow in South Africa. During the past three decades, I have been most fortunate to receive the guidance, teachings and encouragement of some immensely talented and dedicated doctors and professors. It has been a fascinating journey of exploration, the pathway lit by the giants of natural medicine and naturopathic nutrition. More recently, my studies in the field of Functional Medicine have proved immensely helpful and I would like to pay tribute to the genius, courage and dedication of the following specialists who have assisted me enormously in my quest to share the life-changing knowledge contained in this book.

Among them are Dr Boris Chaitow, Debra Waterhouse, Dr Christiane Northrup, Dr Carolyne Dean, Dr Vasant Lad, Dr Mona Lisa Shulz, Dr Loren Cordain, Dr Patrick Vercammen and Dr Ron Grisanti.

I would particularly like to acknowledge the shining inspiration of a truly remarkable doctor who has been a constant source of knowledge, encouragement and inspiration. Dr Ann Lannoye, a Functional Medicine Specialist and member of the Institute of Functional Medicine, has been a most generous and tireless source of knowledge and enthusiasm for the benefits of Functional Medicine. She provided the inspiration to link my nutritional and eating behaviour work with the Functional Diagnostic Medicine and the analysis of Epigenetic Expression. Dr Lannoye's extensive knowledge and scientific rigour have been one of the major cornerstones of our next book about Functional Medicine in which I hope to have Dr Lannoye join me as a contributor and authority.

My functional medicine research and its conclusions have been so fundamental to my understanding of intelligent nutrition, that I undertook studies at the Functional Medicine University in South Carolina. Dr Ron Grisanti has been a most generous provider of case study information in these vitally important subjects.

I am also delighted to announce a series of further projects with Dr Ann Lannoye and Greg Parry PhD, also based in the field of Functional Medicine. We are scheduling a series of international seminars, professional training courses and wellbeing conventions. If you would like to know more go to...

The Paleo Ketogenic Holiday Recipes for Beginners By Beran Parry

Preface

The amazing Paleo Ketogenic Diet did not appear magically overnight or out of thin air. It's the result of many years of research, trial, tribulation and intensive investigation. Despite studying nutrition intensively for over 30 years, I found that I never really reached the permanent weight loss that I wanted. No matter how much weight I lost, I was never really where I wanted to be with my weight.

That has got to be one of the greatest frustrations you can experience when you're trying to get your weight under control. There was usually some initial success but then there'd be some unexpected relapse and this made me realise that there had to be a lot more to real, sustainable weight loss than just following the latest fad or fashion in dieting.

But I never gave up.

If permanent weight loss and becoming a leaner, healthier version of myself was really possible, I was going to find out how to do it. Safely, scientifically and effectively. And that meant more studying, more learning, more experiments, more trials, more creativity, inventing, developing. I approached the problem from every possible angle.

I researched countless scientific studies, the psychological aspects of food choice, the psychology of eating disorders, genetic analysis, functional medicine, naturopathic principles and ayurvedic medicine until a clear picture finally emerged of how to really manage weight issues.

I slowly refined and toned and developed the entire system that has become the Paleo Delicious Diet. It's what you're holding in your hands right now. It's been a long journey but the effort was totally worthwhile. Finally, we've got the smart way for your body to function the way that Nature intended.

My final personal leaner more delicious transformation began seven years ago. After 3 decades of never quite getting there from a weight loss point of view, I decided that enough was enough! It was now or never reaching my real weight loss goals. I knew there was a skinner, more energised, healthier version of me just waiting to get out! With my family's history of weight problems and issues with eating behaviour, plus my own experience of yo-yo dieting and a penchant for delicious food, this was the moment to put my twenty five years of knowledge to the toughest test.

The guinea pig for this extraordinary experiment? You guessed it. Me! I decided it was time to get really serious about my weight loss programme and finally unleash the skinnier new me. I used everything I'd learned, applied the methods I'd been investigating and the pounds slipped away.

And they stayed away. Forever.

I'd finally made all the connections between the different functions of the body and discovered how to eliminate the garbage and toxins from our cells. I'd identified the worst toxins that poison our food. I knew how to create a natural, healthy environment in the gut. I'd discovered how to feed the body with the essential nutrients that would promote natural weight loss and all-round health. In the final phase of my experiment, I learned about the epigenetics revolution from some incredible Doctors of Functional Medicine like Dr Ann Lannoye.

Then I devised a program and over 200 recipes based on using this scientific feedback. During this process of creating a completely effective formula for sustainable weight control a skinnier new me emerged. Finally!

It was a long journey, but I learned so much in every moment of it, and now I am going to share some of the Holiday Recipes with YOU.

The Paleo Ketogenic Holiday Recipes for Beginners By Beran Parry

The Paleo Ketogenic Holiday Recipes for Beginners has already helped countless numbers of people just like you who were looking for a real alternative to all the crazy ideas about weight management.

The Paleo Delicious way of eating enables me to look you in the eye and say I KNOW this WORKS. And now you can enjoy the benefits yourself and become your best body weight and realise your own skinnier potential. And keep it forever!

Let's Start

The Paleo Ketogenic Holiday Recipes for Beginners By Beran Parry

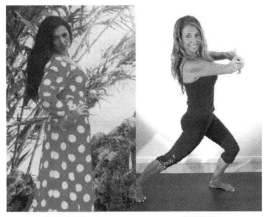

BEFORE   AFTER

My Story

CHAPTER 1

About Beran

As a Bestselling Diet, Nutrition and Fitness Author, with over 20 bestselling Amazon Books to her credit, Beran Parry is passionate about helping YOU permanently improve YOUR Midlife Health, Weight and Wellbeing!

She is fully Certified (Distinction) in Nutritional Therapy, Advanced Diet and Weight Loss, Exercise Physiology and a Pilates Master Teacher.

After helping thousands of women with their Midlife weight and wellbeing challenges, she can to help YOU transform your life forever!

Beran has also trained over 100 Pilates Teachers Worldwide, she is also a Face Pilates Specialist, a Yoga Teacher and has studied with the Top Functional Medicine Doctor in Europe.

Beran's Story

I am a Thyroid Cancer Survivor. I have had a Subtotal Thyroidectomy and been taking synthetic thyroid hormone for over 17 years. I have gained and lost 50 pounds 3 times in my life!

Despite a slow Metabolism, I lost almost 20 pounds during the midlife transition to menopause by simply following my own detailed and precisely targeted research process, a program that has resulted in a complete transformation of my energy levels, my weight, my body shape, my mental and emotional wellbeing and my ability to fully engage and enjoy life!

I had the worst time ever 18 years ago.....

The Paleo Ketogenic Holiday Recipes for Beginners By Beran Parry

In 1999, I had the worst year ever when my mother needed emergency lifesaving open heart surgery, I discovered a thyroid malignancy, I also had major personal relationship challenges and a miscarriage due to non-functioning thyroid and hormone imbalance issues!

Imagine a year where your mother is seriously ill, you get a malignancy diagnosis, you suffer a miscarriage, your marriage is in crisis and you hate your work so much that you feel ill just going to the office every day! That happened to me! The year before I thought everything was wonderful! Fabulous marriage, successful career in finance, although I was having low thyroid symptoms and not realizing it!

A huge feeling of despondency and depression descended on me. I now understand fully what its like to feel utterly devastated with life at every level, my health, my weight, my family's health, my marriage, my job and my emotional framework

Fast forward to 2000 and I really had to sit down and take stock of my life, undergo thyroid removal surgery, deal with low metabolism symptoms, patch up the marriage and admit that my office work was affecting my health!

In 2001, I decided to change my life completely, went back to school to restudy Nutrition, Professional Fitness, Pilates, Yoga and Holistic Therapies and I became a Pilates and Reiki Master.

2002-2012

Things went reasonably well during this period of intense study, research and consulting, but I never quite got to the peak health I wanted, because there were clearly post menopausal issues as well as functional medical issues with inflammatory processes in my gut! and I ended up with quite sensational health challenges post menopause in 2013!

In the past, I suffered from irritable bowel syndrome and in 2013 I had a major healing crisis which affected my nervous system and I was unable to work for 6 months. It became the most challenging yet most exciting educational experience of my life as I discovered functional medicine and created a new eating and supplement plan that healed all my inflammation and nervous system symptoms.

The reason this REALLY excited me was because during my research I discovered through functional medicine that my new way of eating had already helped SO MANY ILL PEOPLE with so many challenging conditions besides obesity. These included auto immune issues, cardio vascular issues, malignancies, hormonal issues, and SO MUCH MORE!

Now I am physically and mentally stronger than I was in my 20's,30's and 40's

My life has been full of challenges and learning experiences on many levels: personally, professionally, through menopause and through many emotional challenges and spiritual quests…… but it has ALL made me SO MUCH STRONGER THAN I EVER WAS!

The Paleo Ketogenic Holiday Recipes for Beginners By Beran Parry

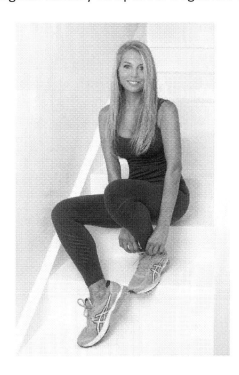

The Paleo Ketogenic Holiday Recipes for Beginners By Beran Parry

My One Major Reoccurring Challenge

I gained over 50 lbs three times in my life during divorce, pregnancy and trans-Atlantic house moves and each time I recovered and lost even more weight to end up at 10 pounds below my teenage weight for the last 10 years!!! During these intense learning experiences, I discovered SO MANY INTERESTING ways I can help you with your quest for excellent wellbeing!

I now live with my best ever body shape, eat a varied, delicious and plentiful diet, exercise and meditate joyously each day and love my life with passion, peace, energy and joy.

I believe that YOU TOO can live YOUR LIFE with passion, peace, energy and joy!

We are going to work together to change behaviors and MAKE THIS HAPPEN FOR YOU!

My passion in life is to dedicate myself to facilitating this same kind of change in anyone who has been through health challenges, particularly around midlife, and I love to inspire real and permanent change and transformation within every person that I work with. It's my raison d'etre

Now, I specialize in helping anyone with Midlife Health and Weight Issues to achieve their personal life and health goals through mindset, habits, exercise and nutritional programs based on functional medicine concepts.

I always advocate holistic wellbeing, healthy lifestyles, the safest and most effective ways for sustained weight loss, Pilates, yoga and body weight training and paleo/keto nutrition.

Daily, I lecture, consult and coach all over the world via skype and in person to empower others to achieve their lifelong health ambitions and turn their goals and dreams into reality

I also run Ultimate Midlife Detox and Boot Camp Retreats around the world to get YOUR Body and Health into its BEST SHAPE EVER!

Now I am dedicating my life and knowledge to help you create YOUR very BEST Wellbeing and Weight Loss Programs

Beran Parry is passionate about helping people around the world reach their wellbeing, fitness, health and weight loss goals;

She is a certified and specialized Nutritional therapist and Advanced Diet and Weight Loss Consultant. She also holds certifications in Exercise Physiology, Pilates, Reiki and EFT.

Beran is also a Master Pilates Trainer, a face Pilates specialist and yoga teacher and a meditation and EFT therapist.

Beran resides in Spain but constantly travels to the USA, UK, Belgium, South Africa and Germany to lecture, consult and lead wellbeing retreats for an international audience. She also consults via skype, telephone, email, video chats and at her local facilities.

The Paleo Ketogenic Holiday Recipes for Beginners By Beran Parry

As a special seasonal gift I would like to offer you my 5 day Paleo Detox at a 50% discount to do before or after the Holiday Season. It contains the following exciting elements

Delicious Recipes,

Stunning Detox Menu's,

Detoxifying Pilates Exercise Videos,

A Daily Detox Face Pilates Program,

Guided Detox Meditations,

FREE Bonus Recipe Books,

FREE Stress Release System

Here is more info and the coupon code

beranparry.com/midlife-fatburn-detox

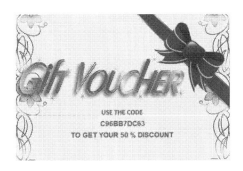

USE THE CODE
C96BB7DC63
TO GET YOUR 50 % DISCOUNT

The Paleo Ketogenic Holiday Recipes for Beginners By Beran Parry

Chapter 2

So Why Can't I Lose Weight? And why can't I keep the weight off?

These are good questions because even champion weight losers often put the weight back on, suffering the seemingly inevitable see-saw effect of cyclical weight loss followed by weight gain. Can we do something to correct this problem? Of course we can! That's exactly what this book is for.

PALEO PARADIGM PYRAMID 1 – YOUR BIGGEST WEIGHT INFLUENCER

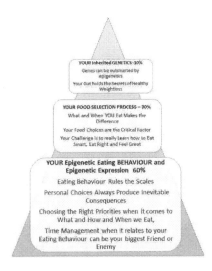

As you might recall from my life story, over the years of battling with weight issues, I tried many, many different methods and diets to lose weight and keep the pounds off. In those early years, with very little useful help or advice, I experienced most of the recurring problems that I bet you're familiar with. Every "weight loss program" was slow and the weight certainly didn't come off very quickly. This was always frustrating and de-motivating. With the SPS weight loss protocol this problem is solved. I lost a total of fifty pounds over the course of eighteen months. When you are losing weight gradually but consistently every day, this keeps your motivation at a very high level. The next problem with every other weight loss system I tried is that I was always hungry and that made me feel pretty miserable most of the time. Does that sound familiar to you? Clearly a better way is needed!

1. Create Good Habits

Willpower - the mantra of the naturally thin. Why willpower alone is overrated

In my Book you will learn about how willpower influences your weight!. This is really amazing info and you need it if you want to lose weight permanently.

Managing your Environment

Before we take a closer look at the mechanics of smart weight loss, we need to think about how we can boost our chances of success by monitoring our environment. The longer you stay on the right track, the more your body will detox and the easier it will feel for you to do the right thing effortlessly all the time.

2. Cravings

Intense hunger. Thin people can never understand this. It's a hard but inescapable fact. An overweight person is physically hungry more often than a naturally thin person.

Eating when your body doesn't need the fuel.

Overweight people are also prone to problems with "emotional eating" or cravings. This hunger might be emotional in origin, but it feels exactly like real physical hunger when you experience it. **Addictions. Are you a food junkie?**

During the 1980s when the arrival of highly processed, cheap cocaine in the form of crack produced an epidemic in drug addiction, researchers were convinced that of all the substances that could cause addiction in humans, food simply could not be classed as addictive. Scientists absolutely refused to consider the possibility that an individual could become addicted to any kind of food. It just wasn't possible.

3. Your Internal Digestion Clock

Eating too late in the evening is a disaster for good digestion and for good sleep. Food and alcohol can disrupt the body's natural digestive cycles and encourage the body to store the food as fat. There's a great deal of interesting modern research on this fascinating topic but the concept is hardly new.

4. Genetics.

There are thousands of diet books, countless weight-loss articles and hundreds of weight loss organisations but we all know about the real problem of losing weight; the fat begins to slip away, we post the good news on Facebook, celebrating the success - and then we see all the good work undone as we put the pounds back on in a very short period of time. Now that is just too frustrating!

The Paleo Ketogenic Holiday Recipes for Beginners By Beran Parry

SUMMARY

Metabolism is the key

Recognising intense hunger and cravings

Creating good habits

Managing your environment

Building support from friends, family and colleagues

Eliminating the villains from the weight loss narrative

The Paleo Ketogenic Holiday Recipes for Beginners By Beran Parry

The Paleo Ketogenic Holiday Recipes for Beginners By Beran Parry

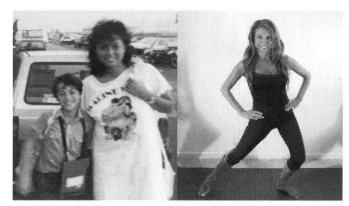

BEFORE   AFTER

Chapter 3

Epigenetics + Long Term Eating Behaviours = Your Present Weight Level

We really believe that knowledge is power and we want you to understand as much about this important subject as possible. Being armed with the best information will strengthen your understanding of how to master your weight issues, take away all that ridiculous and unnecessary guilt about being overweight and prepare you for a newer, happier, skinnier you.

The kind of food we consume every single day, the quality of the food we eat, the eating choices we make all contribute far more to our total health and wellbeing than was ever appreciated before. It's not a question of being pre-programmed by our DNA. We've been bombarded by articles and news items for decades telling us every day that everything in our lives is caused by our genes.

So when we consult the latest reference works in this exciting new area of scientific research, we find that Epigenetics demonstrates the importance of influences which are firmly outside the traditional genetic system. This is the conclusion of Lyle Armstrong, whose research programme is widely respected at the Institute of Genetic Medicine at Newcastle University in the United Kingdom.

The Three Golden Food Rules!... Weight loss is all about insulin

1. Eating Lean...... protein but plenty good quality fat
2. Eat Clean...pure non processed food!
3. Eat Mean.... but only when it comes to sugar and grains!

The Paleo Diet

The Paleo Ketogenic Holiday Recipes for Beginners By Beran Parry

The theory is that many of our current health problems are a result of our modern eating habits. There's been a great deal of publicity surrounding the growing view that we simply haven't evolved to the point where we can safely consume a grain-rich diet. Our distant ancestors in the Old Stone Age or Paleolithic Era consumed a very different diet compared to modern humans because they simply didn't have access to agriculture. That's because agriculture didn't exist. It hadn't been invented. The typical caveman's food was natural, unprocessed, varied, seasonal and a result of labour-intensive, hunter-gathering activities.

The Vegan Option

In a world of unhealthy and even toxic food choices, we shouldn't be surprised that the Vegan diet is associated with lots of positive health benefits. Vegans typically experience lower cholesterol levels, lower blood pressure and less body fat than their meat-eating counterparts. And this might be an important clue about the Vegan success story. If we've been consuming garbage consistently for years and our bodies are suffering from toxic overload, the Vegan diet is a great way to cleanse, heal and restore the digestive system to its natural condition and give our bodies a welcome break from the daily diet of tasty toxins.

Chapter 4

You are now Managing Director of Your Paleo Delicious Life. Inc.

Welcome to Your brand new and exciting career! You are now Managing Director of Your Paleo Delicious Life. Inc. Congratulations. It's simply the Best Job in the Whole World and now it's yours.

Here's what NOT to eat. Cutting out all of these foods and drinks will help you regain your natural, healthy metabolism, reduce systemic inflammation and help you to realise exactly how these foods are truly affecting your weight, fat percentage, health, fitness and every aspect of your life.

The Paleo Delicious Epigenetic Shopping Guide

Being overweight is expensive in every possible way. And it costs far too much in terms of your quality of life. So, it's vitally important to make healthy eating your absolute top priority and there are many of ways for you to maximize your food budget. We'll start with the top priority foods in the Paleo Delicious Diet

The next three items ALL SHARE EQUAL PRIORITY

Priority #1: Protein

Always start at the game, poultry, fish, and eggs section first because the majority of your budget should be spent on high quality animal protein.

- Prime choice:

Always look for organic and/or raised in the wild. Buy whatever's available, and learn how to cook it, if necessary. If you have room in your budget, buy extra and freeze it for later. Go for organic, free-range eggs – they're still one of the cheapest sources of good protein.

- Alternative choice:

If you can't afford organic meat, go for game (ostrich and venison are best), fish and eggs. Chicken is still controversial because we don't know how many hormones and GMO grains are added to chickenfeed these days. Avoid beef and pork since they are too high in fat and usually contain anti-biotics and hormones.

- Never:

Bypass all commercially-raised and/or processed meats (like bacon, sausage and deli meats).

- If you are against consuming animal protein for any reason, you have a great alternative in Hemp Protein Powder

Hemp protein, made from the hemp seed, is a high-fibre protein supplement that can be used to enhance total protein intake for vegans and non-vegans alike. Hemp can be considered a superior protein source due to its above-average digestibility, which also makes it ideal for athletes. When a protein is efficiently digested, it can be deployed more effectively by the body. The digestibility of any given protein is related to the concentrations of its amino acids. A study published in 2010 in the "Journal of Agricultural and Food Chemistry" tested the protein digestibility-corrected amino acid score (PDAAS) -- a rating that determines the bioavailability of a protein -- for various proteins derived from the hemp seed. The results showed that hemp seed proteins have PDAAS values greater than or equal to a variety of grains, nuts and legumes. We're big fans of hemp seed protein because it enhances the immune system and boosts energy levels as well as protecting the kidneys.

Hemp Background

Hemp is a remarkably diverse crop that can be grown for both food and non-food purposes. Hemp seed, which is used to manufacture hemp protein, is composed of approximately 45 percent oil, 35 percent protein and 10 percent carbohydrates. The hemp seed possesses many nutritional benefits, according to Agriculture and Agri-food Canada. In addition to its health benefits, hemp is very environmentally friendly, as it can be grown without the use of fungicides, herbicides and pesticides and it efficiently absorbs carbon dioxide. How many more good reasons do you need to fall in love with hemp seed protein?

Priority #2: Vegetables

Now that you've organised your essential protein supplies, it's time to move on to the vegetables. These are the second tier of your super new plan for effective weight loss and new levels of wellbeing.

- Vegetables are very important in the epigenetic diet plan because they help the body to eliminate toxins and re-balance the microbiome. (By this we mean your gut bacteria). Local produce is the first choice and aim to eat whatever's in season as these veggies are going to be the least expensive and the most nutritious. Choose veggies that are super dense with nutrients. If you have to peel it before eating (or if you don't eat the skin), organic isn't as important. Frozen vegetables can also be an excellent budget-friendly option.
- Fruits: Buy what you can locally (and organically, if possible). If you can't get it locally then it's probably not in season, which means it's not as fresh, not as tasty, and more expensive. Frozen fruits (like berries) are superb, inexpensive alternatives. Add berries and low sugar apples to your shopping list. Bananas, peaches and pineapple should always be consumed in small quantities and we recommend that you eat sparingly grapes, mango, tropical and dried fruit especially during the three-week detox phase.

Priority #3: Healthy Fats

Healthy fats make up the last items on your shopping list. Some of the healthiest fats are also the least expensive and it's always a good idea to keep a good supply of oils, nuts, and seeds at home to help in preparing your super, new delicious meals.

- Canned coconut milk is delicious and provides 72 grams of fat per can. Avocados are a great, all year-round choice too when it comes to sourcing healthy fat.
- Almond milk and other nut-based milks are also recommended but always make sure there is no sugar or salt in the list of ingredients
- Almond or coconut flour make an ideal alternative for baking or for thickening sauces.
- Stock up on coconut oil, extra virgin olive oil, walnut, avocado and hazelnut oil.
- Nuts are a great source of healthy fats but you need to consume them in moderation. Nut butters often contain unnecessary additives to be careful to read the labels. Too many cheaper nuts are salted and roasted in seed or vegetable oils – a less healthy option – so always opt for the raw, natural varieties.

The Paleo Ketogenic Holiday Recipes for Beginners By Beran Parry

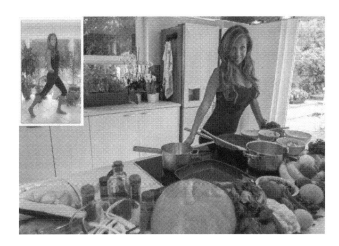

Chapter 5 –

Paleo Budget Tips

There are some really helpful principles you can apply when it comes to shopping for your super-healthy new food choices:

1. Buy seasonal produce. Fruits and vegetables are usually a lot cheaper when they're in season and this can make a major difference to your weekly grocery bill.

2. Don't over-complicate your meals. If you're planning on saving money on your new, healthy food bills, aim for a simple list of ingredients. All you need is a protein, a couple of vegetables, some fat to cook it in and a couple of herbs and spices for flavouring. How simple is that? You can easily tick all the nutritional boxes, eat super-healthy and still save money.

3. A lot of people ignore the benefits of frozen foods when they're a perfect, low cost alternative to fresh or out of season food items. Frozen food broadens your choices and keeps your food bills well within budget.

4. It might not be totally practical to buy 100% organic all the time and we all know that organic food can certainly cost more than the factory-farmed and chemically treated alternatives. Certain foods should always be organic and we've listed a handy reference guide to remind you where the organic emphasis should always be laid;

5. We love eggs and, if you find the organic varieties too expensive, you can always opt for free-range. They're such a versatile, low cost way to include high quality protein in your diet and a fabulous, low cost source of excellent nutrition.

6. Avoid farmed fish wherever possible. We opt for canned Alaskan wild salmon because it's delicious and a very affordable alternative to fresh, wild salmon. When they're in season, fresh mussels are a delicious and popular ingredient for some truly superb dishes.

7. If the full Paleo commitment is going to stretch your budget too much, consider the benefits of following the method for 80% of the time. You'll still notice the difference that healthy food will make to your body and you'll have the satisfaction of moving in the right direction towards a much healthier lifestyle. Some people start the revolution by following the Diet for 50% of the time and that's a whole lot better than using the methods for zero percent of the time! Do what you can.

8. We've mentioned before that budgeting is more often a question of priorities. People will quite happily spend money every month for their cable TV subscription, as if their daily diet of soap operas will somehow benefit their health issues. People fork out money for their monthly cell phone subscriptions yet we complain about the apparent cost of the real food that is the foundation of health, longevity, vitality and absolute wellbeing. It's hard to reconcile the contradiction of spending money on non-essential luxuries and then complaining that real food might be too expensive. It's your life. It's your health. It's your choice.

9. Nuts are a great source of nutrition but they can become expensive when consumed in bulk. Avocados can provide a cost effective alternative way to boost your healthy fat consumption.

10. Meat is a delicious way to enhance your health but if you buy the cheaper cuts, you can tenderise the joints and cuts in a slow cooker that will transform a tougher piece of meat into a succulent dish. It just takes a dash of creativity and a little imagination and you can eat smart on a tight budget.

Ultimately, the real benefits of following the Paleo Diet are revealed in the way the body loses excess weight naturally, in the obvious improvements in health and skin appearance, in the wholly natural boost in energy and vitality levels, in the way we feel. The alternatives to this smart approach to nutrition show up in a list of potentially very unpleasant health problems, diseases that we now know are avoidable. If smart nutrition puts the odds firmly in your favour, you'd have to be nuts to ignore the opportunity to restore the gift of natural health to your body. Once again, it's your body and your choice and, if you're prepared to put a price on your lifelong health and wellbeing, our wish is that you do not value your wellness too cheaply. It's got to be worth every penny you're prepared to invest in your own health.

Chapter 6 –

RECIPES

Holiday Breakfasts (Grain Free)

1. Apple Celebration Dream

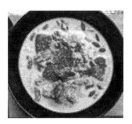

Ingredients:
2 Cup (C) raw walnuts
1 C raw macadamia nuts
2 apples, peeled and diced
1 Tbsp coconut oil
1 Tbsp ground cinnamon
2 C almond milk
1 14 oz can full fat coconut milk

Instructions:
Combine nuts and dates in a food processor until ground into a fine meal, about 1 minute; set aside.
Saute apples over medium heat in coconut oil until lightly browned, about 5 minutes.
Add nut mixture and cinnamon to apples and stir to incorporate, about 1 minute.
Reduce heat to low and add coconut and almond milk.
Stirring occasionally, let mixture cook uncovered until thickened, about 25 minutes.

2. Party Protein Muesli

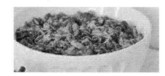

Ingredients:
1 cup unsweetened unsulfured coconut flakes
1 tbsp chopped walnuts
1 tbsp raw almonds (~10)
1 tbsp chocolate chips (dark and sugar free)
1/2 tsp cinnamon
1 cup unsweetened almond milk
1 scoop hemp protein

Instructions:
In a medium bowl layer coconut flakes, walnuts, almonds and chocolate chips.
Sprinkle with cinnamon.
Pour cold almond milk over the muesli and eat with a spoon.

3. Celebratory Apple Almond Coconut Medley

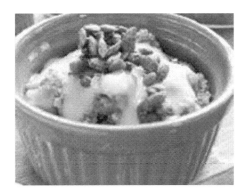

Ingredients:
one-half apple cored and roughly diced
handful of sliced almonds
handful of unsweetened coconut
generous dose of cinnamon
1 pinch of low sodium salt

Instructions:
Pulse in the food processor to desired consistency—smaller is better for the little ones! Serve with almond milk, or creamy coconut milk.

Holiday Egg Meals

4. Latina Eggs with Chilli

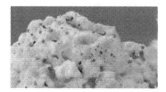

Ingredients:
4 fresh green chillies with skins removed
2 tablespoons (30g or 1 oz) coconut oil
1 small onion, peeled and finely chopped
6 eggs
1/4 cup (62ml or 2 fl oz) coconut milk
low sodium salt to taste

Instructions:
After removing chilli skins, remove and discard seeds and finely chop remaining chilli.
Beat eggs, coconut milk and salt in a bowl and set aside.
Heat oil in a medium size saucepan over a medium heat.
Reduce heat to low and add egg mixture to saucepan and mix well.
Scatter chilies over mixture.
Cook over a low heat until eggs are cooked.
Serves 4. Serve hot.

5. Basil and Walnut Eggs Divine

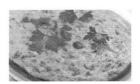

Ingredients:
3 organic eggs
1/2 cup fresh basil, chopped
1/3 cup walnuts, chopped
salt and pepper

Instructions:
Whisk eggs in a bowl then place in a frying pan on medium heat, stirring constantly.

When the eggs are almost cooked, add the basil and continue cooking for a further 1 minute or until eggs are fully cooked.

Add salt and pepper to taste.

Remove from heat and stir in the walnuts before serving.

6. Spicy Sumptious Eggs

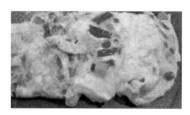

Ingredients:
1 tablespoon extra virgin olive oil
1 red onion, finely chopped
1 medium green pepper, cored, seeded, and finely chopped
1 chilli, seeded and cut into thin strips
3 ripe tomatoes, peeled, seeded, and chopped
Salt and freshly ground black pepper
4 large organic eggs

Instructions:
Heat the olive oil in a large, heavy, preferably nonstick skillet over medium heat.
Add the onion and cook until soft, 6 to 7 minutes.
Add the pepper and chilli and continue cooking until soft, another 4 to 5 minutes.
Add in the tomatoes, and salt and pepper to taste and cook uncovered, over low heat for 10 minutes.
Add the eggs, stirring them into the mixture to distribute.
Cover the skillet and cook until the eggs are set but still fluffy and tender, about 7 to 8 minutes. Divide between 4 plates and serve.

7. Spicy India Egg Party

Ingredients:
3 Eggs
1 Onion, chopped
4 Green Chilli (optional)
1/4 cup Coconut grated
Low sodium Salt as required
1 tblspoon olive oil

Instructions:
Beat the Eggs severely.
Mix chopped onion, rounded green chilli, salt and grated coconuts with eggs.
Heat oil on a medium-low heat, in a pan.
Pour the mixture in the form of pancakes and cook it on the both sides.

8. Spectacular Spinach Omelet

Ingredients:
2 eggs
1.5 cups raw spinach
coconut oil, about 1 tbsp
1/3 c tomatoes and onion salsa (lightly fried in pan)
1 tbsp fresh cilantro

Instructions:
Melt coconut oil on medium in frying pan. Add spinach, cook until mostly wilted. Beat eggs and add to pan.
Flip once the egg sets around the edge. When it's almost done add the salsa on top just to warm it. Move to plate and add cilantro. Serves one.

9. Blushing Blueberry Omelet

Ingredients:
2 eggs
1 tsp. vanilla extract
coconut oil
1/2 c. blueberries
Stevia to taste

Instructions:
Lightly beat two eggs and vanilla extract in a bowl. Heat 6" non-stick pan over medium heat.
While pan is heating, heat half the blueberries in a saucepan until juices flow.
Add coconut oil to non-stick pan and coat evenly.
When thoroughly heated, add egg mixture. Turn once and let sit.
When eggs are about 70% settled, turn again. There should be a nice crispy layer around the side of the pan.
When it starts to separate from the side, add fresh and cooked blueberries to omelet, reserving a few for garnish.
Crispy layer should really be pulling away from pan now.
Use a fork to help fold the omelet over. Slide on to plate, top with reserved blueberry filling, and enjoy!

10. Holiday Supercharger Omelet with Fennel and Dill

Ingredients:
2 tablespoons olive oil, divided
2 cups thinly sliced fresh fennel bulb, fronds chopped and reserved
8 cherry tomatoes
5 large eggs, beaten to blend with 1/4 teaspoon salt and 1/4 teaspoon ground black pepper
1 1/2 tablespoons chopped fresh dill

Instructions:
Add remaining 1 tablespoon oil to same skillet; heat over medium-high heat.
Add beaten eggs and cook until eggs are just set in center, tilting skillet and lifting edges of omelet with spatula to let uncooked portion flow underneath, about 3 minutes.
Top with fennel mixture. Sprinkle dill over.
Using spatula, fold uncovered half of omelet over; slide onto plate.
Garnish with chopped fennel and serve.

11. Outstanding Veggie Omelet

Ingredients:
3 eggs, beaten
1 carrot, matchstick cut
3 scallions, diagonal sliced
1 handful tiny broccoli florets or whatever leftover veggies you have
Bits of leftover cooked turkey
Safflower oil
Low sodium salt

Instructions:
Heat oil in a wok or large cast iron skillet over medium heat, until hot enough to sizzle a drop of water.
Add broccoli and carrots, stir fry 2 min. until soft.
Add cooked turkey, stir fry 1 min. until heated through. Add scallions and eggs, scramble. Add salt to taste. Serve.

12. Spicy Spinach Bake

Ingredients:
6 eggs
1 bunch fresh spinach chopped (a box of frozen will do if you do not have fresh)
1/2 tsp hot pepper flakes
Olive oil
Low sodium Salt and pepper

Instructions:
Scramble the eggs in a bowl. Add the spinach, low sodium salt and pepper.
Scramble together. Heat a large non-stick skillet with about 1/2 cup olive oil.
When the oil is hot put the hot pepper flakes in then pour the mixture in. When it starts to cook on the bottom, flip it over
Take it out when it is medium scrambled. Let cool and eat.

13. Post Thanksgiving Veggie Hash With Eggs

Ingredients:
2 tablespoon extra virgin olive oil
2 garlic cloves, minced
1/4 cup sweet white onion, chopped
1 cup yellow squash, chopped
1/2 cup mushroom, sliced
Low sodium salt and pepper
1 cup cherry tomatoes, halved
1 cup fresh spinach, chopped
4 eggs, poached or cooked any style
You can substitute the squash with whatever vegetables you have

Instructions:
Heat large non-stick skillet over medium heat. Add olive oil to pan.
Add garlic and onion and saute for 2 minutes, then add chopped squash or your favorite vegetable, cook for 2 more minutes, then add mushrooms. Cook for 5-minutes or until almost compete.
At this point add low sodium salt and pepper, then add tomatoes and spinach and cook until spinach wilts. Drain well before plating.
While finishing this prepare eggs to your liking in another pan.
To serve, drained hash mixture to and then add to individual plates. On top of hash add 2 cooked eggs per person.

14. Spectacular Eggie Salsa

Ingredients:
2 pounds fresh ripe tomatoes, peeled and coarsely chopped
2 to 3 serrano or jalapeño chiles, seeded for a milder sauce, and chopped
2 garlic cloves, peeled, halved, green shoots removed
1/2 small onion, chopped
2 tablespoons oil
Low sodium salt to taste
4 to 8 eggs (to taste)
Chopped cilantro for garnish

Instructions:
Place the tomatoes, chiles, garlic and onion in a blender and puree, retaining a bit of texture.
Heat 1 tablespoon of the oil over high heat in a large, heavy nonstick skillet, until a drop of puree will sizzle when it hits the pan.
Add the puree and cook, stirring, for four to ten minutes, until the sauce thickens, darkens and leaves a trough when you run a spoon down the middle of the pan. It should just begin to stick to the pan.
Season to taste with salt, and remove from the heat. Keep warm while you fry the eggs.
Warm four plates. Fry the eggs in a heavy skillet over medium-high heat.
Use the remaining tablespoon of oil if necessary. Cook them sunny side up, until the whites are solid but the yolks still runny.
Season with salt and pepper, and turn off the heat. Place one or two fried eggs on each plate.
Spoon the hot salsa over the whites of the eggs, leaving the yolks exposed if possible. Sprinkle with cilantro and serve.

15. Mushrooms, Eggs and Onion Bonanza

Ingredients:
1 medium onion, finely diced
1/4 cup coconut oil
10-12 medium white mushrooms, finely chopped
12 hard boiled eggs, peeled and finely chopped
Freshly ground black pepper to taste

Instructions:
Saute the onion in coconut oil until golden brown.
Add the mushrooms and saute another 5 minutes or so, stirring frequently, until mushrooms are softened and turned dark.
Remove from heat and let cool.
Mix together with the eggs and pepper. Chill until ready to serve.

16. Celebratory Avocado and Shrimp Omelet

Ingredients:
6 eggs
2 Tbsp. chopped parsley
2 Tbsp. lemon juice, divided
1/4 tsp. salt
1/8 tsp. cayenne pepper
1 large* ripe avocado, diced
1 1/2 Tbsp. avocado oil
3 oz. bay shrimp
3 parsley sprigs

Instructions:
Beat together eggs, parsley, 3/4 of the lemon juice, salt, and cayenne pepper; reserve.
Gently toss avocado with remaining lemon juice; reserve.
Heat oil in an omelet pan. (Use a large omelet pan for four or more servings.)
Pour egg mixture into pan.
Cook over medium heat, lifting edges and tilting pan to allow uncooked egg to run under, until set but still moist on top.
Scatter reserved avocado and shrimp over omelet.
Fold omelet in half; heat another minute or two.
Slide onto a warmed serving plate; garnish with parsley sprigs.
To serve, cut omelet into wedges.

17. Delish Veggie Breakfast Peppers

Ingredients:
2 bell peppers – your choice of color
4 eggs
1 cup white mushrooms
1 cup broccoli
¼ tsp cayenne pepper
low sodium salt and pepper, to taste

Instructions:
Preheat oven to 375 degrees Fahrenheit.
Dice up your vegetables of choice.
In a medium sized bowl, mix eggs, low sodium salt, pepper, cayenne pepper, and vegetables.
Cut peppers into equal halves. A tip:
Core the peppers so that they're clean enough to add the filling.
Pour a quarter of the egg / vegetable mix into each pepper half, adding more vegetables to the top to fill in any empty space.
Place on baking sheet and cook approximately 35 minutes.

18. Breakfast Mexicana Fiesta

Ingredients:
For the tortillas:
2 eggs
2 egg whites
1/2 cup water
4 tsp ground flaxseed
Pinch of low sodium salt

For the filling:
1 avocado, diced
1/4 cup red bell pepper, finely diced
1/4 cup onion, finely diced
1/4 cup baked cod or other protein
Handful of spinach leaves
1 tsp coconut oil

Instructions:
In a small bowl, whisk together the ingredients for the tortilla. Preheat the oven
Heat a 10-inch non-stick skillet over medium heat and coat well with coconut oil spray.
Pour half of the tortilla mixture into the pan and swirl to evenly distribute.
Using a metal spatula, loosen the edges of the tortilla from the pan.
Cook a couple of minutes until golden brown on the bottom, and then carefully slide the spatula under the tortilla to loosen it from the bottom of the pan. Do not flip yet.
Place the pan under the broiler for 3-4 minutes until the tortilla gets a little bubbly.
Remove the tortilla from the pan, setting on a piece of aluminum foil. Repeat with other half of tortilla mixture.
After the tortillas are done broiling, preheat the oven to 400 degrees F. In a separate small pan, heat the coconut oil over medium heat.
Add the onions and peppers and sauté for 5-8 minutes, until soft. Add the spinach into the pan and wilt.
Place all of the fillings down the center of the tortillas and wrap tightly. Place into the oven for 5-8 minutes to set. It's so delish!

19. Zucchini Party Casserole

Ingredients:
3 large zucchini
1/2 red onion, chopped
1/2 cup mushrooms
5 eggs
1 tsp low sodium salt
Freshly ground black pepper, to taste

Instructions:
Preheat oven to 375 degrees F..
Grate all of the zucchini and put into a large bowl.
In a separate bowl, beat the eggs with low sodium salt and pepper.
Combine all of the ingredients, in the large bowl and mix together. You want to have enough eggs to coat the whole mixture.
Warm about a 1/2 tablespoon of olive oil in the skillet over medium heat.
Add the zucchini mixture into the pan. Cover and cook about 5 minutes until the eggs start to set on the bottom.
Transfer to the oven and bake for 12-15 minutes, until the eggs are firm. Remove and let rest for 5-10 minutes, then serve.

20. Blueberry Nut Casserole

Ingredients:
Crush one cup almonds, walnuts and pecans with one teaspoon olive oil and bake in the oven at 200degrees for 20 minutes
2 cups frozen blueberries
5 eggs
1 cup almond milk
Stevia to taste
1 tsp vanilla extract
1 tsp cinnamon
Pinch of nutmeg

Instructions:
Preheat the oven to 350 degrees F. Grease an 8x8-inch baking dish with coconut oil spray. Place the nut crust and blueberries into the dish.
Whisk together the eggs, almond milk, stevia, vanilla, and cinnamon in a medium bowl.
Pour the egg mixture over the crust and blueberries. Lightly stir to coat.
Bake for 35-45 minutes. Remove from the oven and allow the casserole to rest for 15 minutes before serving.

The Paleo Ketogenic Holiday Recipes for Beginners By Beran Parry

Holiday Main Course (Lunch or Dinner)

Turkey and Chicken Meals

21. Spicy Holiday Turkey Stir Fry

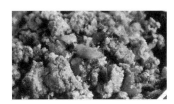

Ingredients:
2 lbs. boneless skinless chicken or turkey breasts, cut into 1-inch slices
2 tbsp coconut oil
1 tsp cumin seeds
1/2 each green, red, and orange bell pepper, thinly sliced
1 tsp garam masala
2 tsp freshly ground pepper
low sodium salt, to taste
Scallions, for garnish

For the marinade:
1/2 cup coconut cream
1 clove garlic, minced
1 tsp ginger, minced
1 tbsp freshly ground pepper
2 tsp low sodium salt
1/4 tsp turmeric

Instructions:
Place all of the marinade ingredients into a Ziploc bag. Add the chicken, close the bag, and shake to coat.
Marinate in the refrigerator for at least 30 minutes, or up to 6 hours.
In a wok or large sauté pan, melt the coconut oil over medium-high heat. Add the cumin seeds and cook for 2-3 minutes. Add the marinated chicken and let cook for 5 minutes. Stir the chicken until it begins to brown, and then add the peppers, garam masala, and freshly ground pepper.
Sprinkle with low sodium salt. Cook for 4-5 minutes, stirring regularly, or until the bell pepper is cooked to desired doneness. Serve hot.

22. Party Roasted Lemon Herb Chicken

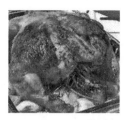

Ingredients:
12 total pieces bone-in chicken thighs and legs
1 medium onion, thinly sliced
1 tbsp dried rosemary
1 tsp dried thyme
1 lemon, sliced thin
1 orange, sliced thin

For the marinade:
5 tbsp extra virgin olive oil
6 cloves garlic, minced
Stevia to taste
Juice of 1 lemon
Juice of 1 orange
1 tbsp Italian seasoning – salt free
1 tsp onion powder
Dash of red pepper flakes
low sodium salt and freshly ground pepper, to taste

Instructions:
Whisk together all of the marinade ingredients in a small bowl. Place the chicken in a baking dish (or a large Ziploc bag) and pour the marinade over it. Marinate for 3 hours to overnight.
Preheat the oven to 400 degrees F. Place the chicken in a baking dish and arrange with the onion, orange, and lemon slices.
Sprinkle with thyme, rosemary, low sodium salt and pepper. Cover with aluminum foil and bake for 30 minutes.
Remove the foil, baste the chicken, and bake for another 30 minutes uncovered, until the chicken is cooked through.

23. Roasted and Filled Bell Peppers Feast

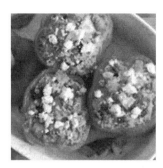

Ingredients:
5 large bell peppers
1 tbsp coconut oil
1/2 large onion, diced
1 tsp dried oregano
1/2 tsp low sodium salt
1 lb. ground turkey
1 large zucchini, halved and diced
3 tbsp tomato paste
Freshly ground black pepper, to taste
Fresh parsley, for serving

Instructions:
Preheat the oven to 350 degrees F. Coat a small baking dish with coconut oil spray. Bring a large pot of water to a boil. Cut the stems and very top of the peppers off, removing the seeds. Place in boiling water for 4-5 minutes. Remove from the water and drain face-down on a paper towel.

Heat the coconut oil in a large nonstick pan over medium heat. Add in the onion. Sauté for 3-4 minutes until the onion begins to soften. Stir in the ground turkey, oregano, low sodium salt, and pepper and cook until turkey is browned.

Add the zucchini to the skillet as the turkey finishes cooking. Cook everything together until the zucchini is soft, and then drain any juices from the pan.

Remove the pan from heat and stir in the tomato paste. Bake for 15 minutes.

24. Party Pasta and Turkey Bolognaise

Ingredients:
4 medium zucchini

For the sauce:
1 lb ground turkey
1 small onion, chopped
4 cloves garlic, minced
1 tbsp coconut oil
1 tomato, chopped
1/2 jar of tomato sauce
1 tbsp Italian seasoning
low sodium salt and pepper to taste
Fresh basil, for garnish

Instructions:
Use a julienne peeler to slice the zucchini into noodles, stopping when you reach the seeds. Set aside.
If cooking zucchini noodles, simply add to a skillet and sauté over medium heat for 4-5 minutes.
Melt coconut oil in a large skillet over medium heat. Add chopped onion and garlic and cook for 4-5 minutes.
Add ground turkey and brown the meat, stirring occasionally. Season with low sodium salt and pepper.
Add the chopped tomato, tomato sauce, and Italian seasoning and stir to combine. Simmer on low heat, stirring occasionally.
Add the sauce to the noodles and ENJOY.

25. Thanksgiving Turkey Spaghetti Squash Boats

Ingredients:
1 medium spaghetti squash or 2 small spaghetti squash
1 1/2 lbs. Turkey mashed
1 yellow onion, diced
4 cloves garlic, minced
1 bunch kale
3 tbsp extra virgin olive oil, plus more for drizzling
low sodium salt and pepper
2 tbsp pine nuts, roasted
2 tbsp fresh parsley, chopped

Instructions:
Preheat the oven to 400 degrees F. Place squash in the microwave for 3-4 minutes to soften. Using a sharp knife cut the squash in half lengthwise. Scoop out the seeds and discard.

Place the halves, with the cut side up, on a rimmed baking sheet. Drizzle with olive oil and sprinkle with low sodium salt and pepper.

Roast in the oven for 45-50 minutes, until you can poke the squash easily with a fork. Let cool until you can handle it safely.

Meanwhile, prepare the kale by removing the center stems and either tearing or cutting up the leaves. Heat the olive oil in a large skillet over medium heat.

Add the onion and garlic and sauté for 4-5 minutes. Add the turkey. Cook for 10-12 minutes, stirring regularly, until the turkey is browned and cooked through.

Add the kale and stir. Cook for a few minutes more to wilt the kale. Remove from heat and set aside.

Once cooled, scrape the insides of the spaghetti squash with a fork to shred the squash into strands. Transfer the strands into the skillet with the turkey and toss to combine.

Season to taste with low sodium salt and pepper. Divide the mixture among the squash shells, and then top with pine nuts and parsley to serve.

26. Tantalizing Turkey Party Stir-fry

Ingredients:
2 bell peppers, sliced
1 cup broccoli florets
2 cooked and shredded turkey breasts
1/4 teaspoon chili powder
low sodium salt and pepper to taste
1 tablespoon coconut oil for frying

Instructions:
Add 1 tablespoon coconut oil into a frying pan on a medium heat.
Place the sliced bell peppers into the frying pan.
After the bell peppers soften, add in the cooked turkey meat.
Add in the chili powder, low sodium salt and pepper.
Mix well and stir-fry for a few more minutes.

27. Sexy Turkey Scramble

Ingredients:
1 pound ground turkey
2 medium yellow onions
2 bell peppers (any color)
2 medium squash or zucchini
1 large hand-full of fresh spinach (2-3 ounces)
Spices to taste: I used about 1 tablespoon each of: cumin, chili powder, garlic powder, low sodium salt, and fresh cilantro

Instructions:
Brown the turkey until well cooked in a large skillet or wok over medium high heat.
Remove and add thinly sliced onions, peppers, squash/zucchini to the pan and saute, stirring constantly, until starting to soften.
Return turkey to pan and add fresh spinach.
Spice to taste and continue to cook until spinach is wilted.
Remove and serve with any desired toppings.

28. Chicken Fennel Feast

Ingredients:
3 chicken breasts or the meat from 1 whole roasted chicken
2 tablespoons coconut oil
1 onion
1 bulb of fennel
1 teaspoon each of low sodium salt, pepper, garlic powder and basil

Instructions:
Stovetop:
Cut the chicken into bite sized pieces. If chicken is raw, heat butter/coconut oil in large skillet or wok until melted.
Add chicken and cook on medium/high heat until chicken is cooked through. (If chicken is pre-cooked, cook the vegetables first then add chicken)
While cooking, cut the onion into bite sized pieces (1/2 inch) and thinly slice the fennel bulb into thin slivers.
Add all to skillet or wok, add spices and continue sautéing until all are cooked through and fragrant.
This will take approximately 10-12 minutes.

Holiday Starter Course - Fish

29. Tempting Thai Baked Fish with Squash Noodles

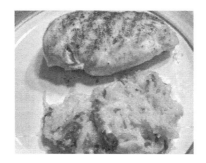

Ingredients:
1 medium spaghetti squash
Extra virgin olive oil, for drizzling
low sodium salt and pepper
1 tbsp coconut oil
1/2 large onion, finely chopped
1 head broccoli, de-stemmed and cut into florets
2 heads baby bok choy, sliced into 1-inch strips
4 scallions, sliced
1/4 tsp red pepper flakes
1/3 cup cashews, toasted and chopped

For the Sauce:
1 tsp lime juice
1/2-inch piece fresh ginger, peeled and minced
1 clove garlic, minced
1/2 tsp red wine vinegar
3 tbsp almond butter
3 tbsp coconut milk

For the Fish:
2 whole fish fillets...use cod or any good quality white fish

Instructions:

Preheat the oven to 400 degrees F. Place squash in the microwave for 3-4 minutes to soften. Using a sharp knife, cut the squash in half lengthwise. Scoop out the seeds and discard. Place the halves, with the cut side up, on a rimmed baking sheet. Drizzle with olive oil and sprinkle with low sodium salt and pepper. Roast in the oven for 45-50 minutes, until you can poke the squash easily with a fork. Let cool until you can handle it safely. Then scrape the insides with a fork to shred the squash into strands.

While the squash cooks, make the sauce. Combine the lime juice, ginger, garlic, and red wine vinegar in a blender or food processor until smooth. Add the almond butter and coconut milk and blend until completely combined. Adjust the levels of almond butter and coconut milk to reach desired level of creaminess.

Melt the coconut oil in a large pan over medium heat. Add the onion and cook for 5-6 minutes until translucent. Add the broccoli and sauté for 8-10 minutes, until just tender. Then stir in the bok choy and cook for 3-4 minutes until wilted. Lastly add the cooked spaghetti squash into the pan and stir to combine.

To assemble, top the spaghetti squash mixture with the scallions and cilantro. Sprinkle with roasted cashews and drizzle with Thai sauce.

Place the whole fish under the grill at 200 degrees for 25 minutes topped with a tablespoon of olive oil, fresh pressed garlic (one clove) and cayenne pepper to taste.

Finnish off the fish with a squirt of lemon juice to taste.

30. Superior Salmon with Lemon and Thyme OR Use any White fish

Ingredients:
32 oz piece of salmon or any fresh white fish
1 lemon, sliced thin
1 tbsp capers
low sodium salt and freshly ground pepper
1 tbsp fresh thyme
Olive oil

Instructions:
Line a rimmed baking sheet with parchment paper and place salmon, skin side down, on the prepared baking sheet. Season salmon with low sodium salt and pepper. Arrange capers on the salmon, and top with sliced lemon and thyme. Place baking sheet in a cold oven, then turn heat to 400 degrees F. Bake for 25 minutes. Serve immediately.

31. Party Delish Baked dill Salmon

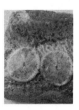

Ingredients:
2 6-oz. salmon fillets
2 zucchini, halved lengthwise and thinly sliced
1/4 red onion, thinly sliced
1 tsp fresh dill, chopped
2 slices lemon
1 tbsp fresh lemon juice
Extra virgin olive oil, for drizzling
low sodium salt and freshly
ground pepper

Instructions:
Preheat the oven to 350 degrees F. Prepare a baking tray
Place half of the zucchini, red onion, dill, and one lemon slice. Drizzle with olive oil and sprinkle with low sodium salt and pepper. Place a salmon fillet on top and drizzle with the lemon juice. Season with low sodium salt and pepper. Repeat with the remaining ingredients.
Bake for 15-20 minutes until the salmon is opaque.

32. Holiday Salmon in Herb Crust

Ingredients:
2 salmon fillets (approx. 300g)
1 small onion, peeled and quartered
2 garlic cloves, peeled
1 sprig lemongrass, coarsely chopped
2 cm piece of ginger root, peeled
1 red chili pepper

Instructions:
Line a rimmed baking sheet with parchment paper and place salmon, skin side down, on the prepared baking sheet.
Generously season salmon with low sodium salt and pepper and top with sliced lemon and thyme.
Place baking sheet in a cold oven, then turn heat to 400 degrees F. Bake for 25 minutes.
Add lemon juice and serve immediately.

33. Salmon Mustard Delish

Ingredients:
4 tsp mustard seed
1/2 tsp garlic powder
1/4 tsp low sodium salt
1/4 tsp black pepper
1/4 tsp dried dill
1 1/2 lb salmon

Instructions:
Preheat oven to 200 degrees Celsius. (390 F)
Start by making the herb crust: combine the onion, garlic, lemongrass, ginger in the smallest bowl of a food processor
Process into a coarse paste.
Put the salmon fillets in an oven dish and spread the herb paste on top.
Bake for approx. 12-15 minutes until done, depending on the thickness of your fillets.
Serve with veggies of your choice and enjoy!

34. Garlic Lemon Shrimp Bonanza

Ingredients:
1 lb shrimp, deveined
3-4 cloves of garlic, chopped
1/2 fresh lemon juice
3 tbsp olive oil
1/8 of low sodium salt
Fresh ground pepper (to taste)
1 tbsp fresh parsley, chopped for garnish

Instructions:
Preheat the broiler, if using. Heat the olive oil in a heavy skillet over medium-low heat.
 Add the garlic and saute, stirring frequently, for about five minutes, until the garlic is softened but not browned.
Add the shrimp, raise the heat to medium high, and sprinkle with low sodium salt, pepper, paprika, and red pepper.
Cook for three minutes on each side or until the shrimp are completely opaque. Serve hot.

35. Celebratory Courgette Pesto and Shrimp

Ingredients:
For the Pesto Sauce:
A ton of Basil
Minced Garlic
Pine Nuts
low sodium salt & Pepper

For the Zinguine:
1 Small Zucchini
low sodium salt & Pepper to taste

For the Shrimp:
Shrimp (peeled & de-veined)

Instructions:
Heat pan to medium-high heat.
Add ghee and garlic. Saute for about a minute.
Add shrimp. Saute for about a minute on each side.
Add low sodium salt, pepper and lemon juice. Saute for another minute or so.
Remove from heat and dish onto a plate or bowl.

36. Cheeky Curry Shrimp

Ingredients:
1 lb raw, peeled, tail on shrimp
2 tsp curry powder
1 tsp garlic powder
1 tsp ground coriander
1/2 tsp ground ginger
low sodium salt and black pepper to taste

Instructions:
In a medium bowl, mix the coconut cream, and lemon juice until combined.
Add the shrimp, tomato, cucumbers, capers, and spices.
Mix until everything is incorporated. Add additional low sodium salt and pepper to taste. Serve in endive leaves.

37. Sexy Shrimp on Sticks

Ingredients:
1/2 lb shrimp, peeled and deveined
1/4 cup coconut milk
1 tsp fish sauce
6 gloves garlic, chopped
1/4 tsp each turmeric, cumin, low sodium salt

Instructions:
Heat olive oil in a large pan over medium heat. Add garlic and spices
Add shrimp and coconut last. Low sodium salt and pepper to taste and serve with a fresh squeeze of lemon.
Serve along side your choice of vegetable or fried cauliflower rice.

Holiday Starter Salad – Animal Protein

38. Delicious Slaw

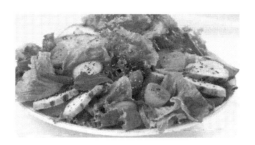

Ingredients:
1/2 head of cabbage   (mix purple and white)
3 or 4 carrots
1 onion
3 tablespoons walnut oil
1 egg beaten
Stevia and low sodium salt to taste
1 Tbsp. fresh lemon juice
pepper to taste

Instructions:
Grate cabbage, carrots and onion and mix together.
Make dressing by mixing
beaten egg, walnut oil, lemon juice, and seasonings.
Chill and serve.

39. Tastylicious Cabbage Salad

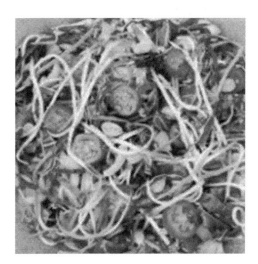

Ingredients:
1 small head purple cabbage, grated
1 small head romaine lettuce, grated
2 medium carrots, julienned
1/2 cup tahini dressing (recipe below)

For dressing:
1/2 cup raw tahini
1/2 cup freshly squeezed lemon juice
2 tablespoons olive oil
1 teaspoon sea salt

Instructions:
Mix the dressing ingredient in a blender until you get a smooth puree then set aside.
***You can save and store excess dressing up to 3 days in the fridge.
Combine the cabbage, lettuce, and carrots in a large bowl, toss with your dressing, and serve immediately.
You can also top it with avocado or tomatoes.
Enjoy!

40. Chicken Basil Avo Salad

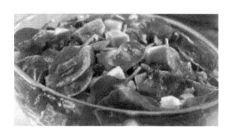

Ingredients:
2 boneless, skinless chicken breasts (organic, cooked and shredded)
1/2 cup fresh basil leaves, stems removed
1 cup sliced cherry tomatoes
2 small or 1 large ripe avocado, pits and skin removed
2 Tbsp. extra virgin olive oil
1/2 tsp. low sodium salt (or more to taste)
1/8 tsp. ground black pepper (or more to taste)

Instructions:
Place the cooked shredded chicken in a medium sized mixing bowl.
Place the basil, avocado, olive oil, low sodium salt and ground black pepper in a food processor and blend until smooth. You may need to scrape the sides a couple times to incorporate.
Pour the avocado and basil mixture into the mixing bowl with the shredded chicken and tomatoes and toss well to coat.
Taste and add additional low sodium salt and ground black pepper if desired. Keep in the fridge until ready to serve.

41. Thanksgiving Turkey Taco Salad

Ingredients:
1/2 lbs (ish) leftover turkey, cooked and chopped
1 1/2 Tbsp taco seasoning (recipe follows)
1 tblsp. coconut or olive oil and 1 tblsp rice vinegar
1/4 c. water
Shredded lettuce

Optional Toppings - sliced olives, tomatoes, red onion, avocado, bell peppers, crushed sweet potato chips

Taco Seasoning:
Mix together, 4 Tbsp. chili powder, 1 tsp each garlic powder, onion powder, and oregano, 2 tsp each paprika and cumin, 4 tsp low sodium salt, and 1/8-1/4 tsp red pepper flakes.

Instructions:
In a skillet, heat 1 teaspoon oil and add in chicken - I like to fry it for a minute to give some extra flavor. Add in water and taco seasoning, let simmer until liquid is gone.
Meanwhile, shred, chop, and dice all your toppings.
Assemble, lettuce, optional toppings, chicken, leftover oil and vinegar dressing, and crushed chips.

42. Macadamia Chicken Salad

Ingredients:
1lb organic chicken breast
1tsp macadamia nut oil, or oil of choice
few pinches of low sodium salt and pepper
1/2 cup macadamia nuts, chopped
1/2 cup diced celery
2 tbsp julienned basil
1 tablespoon olive oil and 2 teaspoons rice vinegar
1 tbsp lemon juice

Instructions:
Preheat oven to 350. Place chicken breasts on sheet tray, drizzle will oil and a pinch of low sodium salt and pepper. Bake for about 35 minutes until cooked through. Remove from oven and let cool.
In a large bowl shred chicken. Add nuts, celery, basil, dressing, and a pinch of low sodium salt and pepper. Gently stir until combined. Eat!

43. Turkey Sprouts Salad

Ingredients:
1/2 pound of brussels sprouts (2-ish cups once sliced)
1/2 cup chopped almonds
2 turkey breasts, chopped
1/2 white onion, finely diced

Vinaigrette:
2 TBSP Apple Cider Vinegar
1 TBSP quality mustard powder
1 TBSP avocado oil
Stevia to taste
1/2 tsp low sodium salt
few grinds of black pepper

Instructions:
Cut the brussels sprouts in half and thinly slice. Chop the half cup of almonds. Finely dice the white onion. Scallions would work too if you prefer a more mild onion flavor... though the white did not overpower.
Remove the breasts and chop into bite-sized pieces. Combine all of these ingredients into a large bowl and gently toss the Brussels sprouts salad.
Whipping up the vinaigrette takes seconds. Add all ingredients to a small bowl and whisk until smooth. Pour over the Brussels sprouts salad and toss to bring together.

44. Avocado Tuna Salad

Ingredients:
2 tins high quality albacore tuna
1 avocado
1/4 of an onion, chopped
juice of 1/2 a lime
2 Tbsp cilantro (or sub basil if you prefer)
some low sodium salt and pepper, to taste

Instructions:
Shred the tuna.
Add all of the other ingredients and mix.

45. Asian Aspiration Salad

Ingredients:
1 red bell pepper, sliced
1 large carrot, cut into matchsticks
1 cucumber, halved lengthwise and sliced

Optional:
fresh ginger juice and rice vinegar
2 boiled eggs

Instructions:
Mix ingredients and Serve.

46. Creamy Carrot Salad

Ingredients:
1 pound carrots - shredded
20 ounces crushed pineapple -- drained
8 ounces Coconut milk
3/4 cup flaked coconut
Stevia to taste
Shredded turkey one breast

Instructions:
Combine all ingredients, tossing well. Cover and chill.

47. Tasty Tuna Stuffed Tomato

Ingredients:
2 large tomatoes
Lettuce leaves (optional)
2 (5 or 6 oz.) cans wild albacore tuna
6 Tbsp. olive oil and 1 tablespoon rice vinegar
1 stalk celery, chopped
1/2 small onion, chopped
1/4 tsp. low sodium salt
1/4 tsp. ground black pepper

Instructions:
Wash and dry the tomatoes and remove any stem. You can either slice off the top part of the tomatoes and hollow them out, or cut each tomato into wedges, making sure to only cut down to about 1/2 inch before you get to the bottom of the tomato.
Arrange the tomatoes on a plate on top of lettuce leaves (optional).
Combine the remaining ingredients in a mixing bowl and add additional low sodium salt and/or pepper if desired. Spoon into the tomatoes and serve.

Holiday Desserts

48. Rose Banana Delicious Brownies

Ingredients:
2 red beets, cooked
2 bananas
2 eggs
1/2 cup unsweetened cacao powder
1/3 cup almond flour
1 tsp baking powder
3 tablespoons crushed mixed nuts
Stevia to taste

Instructions:
Combine all ingredients in a food processor, and blend until smooth.
Stir in the nut bits
Pour into a well-greased pan about 8x8 inches
Bake at 325 for about 40 minutes.

49. Secret Sumptious Brownies

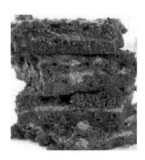

Ingredients:
1 c. raw almonds
1/2 c. raw cashews
4-5 Tbs. cocoa powder
1 Tbs. cashew butter
Stevia to taste

Instructions:
Combine all ingredients in the food processor.
Whir until somewhat smooth.
Press into 8×8" glass baking dish.
Chill until ready to serve.

50. Choco-coco Brownies

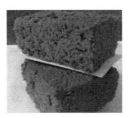

Ingredients:
6 Tablespoons of coconut oil
6 ounces of Sugar free Chocolate
4 Tablespoons of Packed Coconut Flour (20g)
¼ cup of Unsweetened Cocoa Powder (30g)
2 Eggs
½ teaspoon of Baking Soda
¼ teaspoon of low sodium salt
Extra coconut oil for pan greasing
Stevia to taste

Instructions:
Preheat the oven to 350F. Grease an 8x8 baking pan and line with parchment paper.
Ensure eggs are at room temperature. You may run them under warm water for about 10 seconds while shelled.
Gently melt the semisweet chocolate and oil in a double boiler. You may use the microwave at 50% heat at 30 second intervals with intermittent stirring.
Stir in unsweetened cocoa powder.
Sift together the superfine coconut flour, baking soda, stevia and low sodium salt.
Beat the eggs and add the dry ingredients. Beat until combined
Add the rest of the wet ingredients and beat until incorporated.
Pour the batter into the lined 8x8 pan.
Bake for 25-30 minutes at 350F until a toothpick inserted into the center of the batter comes out clean.
When done, remove from the oven and let cool in the pan for at least 15 minutes.

51. Coco – Walnut Brownie Bites

Ingredients:
2/3 cup raw walnut halves and pieces
1/3 cup unsweetened cocoa powder
1 tablespoon vanilla extract
1 to 2 tablespoons coconut milk
2/3 cups shredded unsweetened coconut

Instructions:
Pulse coconut in food processor for 30 seconds to a minute to form coconut crumbs. Remove from food processor and set aside.
Add unsweetened cocoa powder and walnuts to food processor, blend until walnuts become fine crumbs, but do not over process or you will get some kind of chocolate walnut butter.
Place in the food processor the cocoa walnut crumbs. Add vanilla. Process until mixture starts to combine.
Add coconut milk. You will know the consistency is right when the dough combines into a ball in the middle of the food processor.
If dough is too runny add a tablespoon or more cocoa powder to bring it back to a dough like state.
Transfer dough to a bowl and cover with plastic wrap. Refrigerate for at least 2 hours. Cold dough is much easier to work with. I left my dough in the fridge over night. You could put it in the freezer if you need to speed the process up.
Roll the dough balls in coconut crumbs, pressing the crumbs gently into the ball. Continue until all dough is gone.

52. Party Peach and Almond Cake

Ingredients:
2 whole peaches
300g almond meal
6 eggs
Stevia to taste
1 tsp baking soda

Instructions:
Cover the peaches in water in a saucepan and boil for about 2 hours.
Preheat the oven to 180 degrees Celsius and line the bottom of a 24cm pan with baking paper.
Lightly beat the eggs.
Blend the eggs and peaches (quarter them first) thoroughly in a food processor.
Add the rest of the ingredients to the food processor, again blending thoroughly.
Pour mixture into the lined tin and bake for roughly an hour.

53. Fetching Fudge

Ingredients:
1 cup coconut butter
1/4 cup coconut oil
1/4 cup cocoa
1/4 cup cocoa powder + 1 Tbsp
Stevia to taste
1 tsp vanilla

Instructions:
In the pot, gently melt the cocoa butter on low (number 2)
When it is half melted add the butter, the coconut oil and the coconut spread and gently mix with the whisk as it melts
Add vanilla, and stevia and whisk in well
Add the cocoa powder and whisk in well
Be sure to take the pot off the heat when the fat is melted and keep whisking until it is smooth and all the lumps are out — you don't want to overheat this
Pour into the 8 x 8 pan that is lined with parchment paper
Refrigerate for 1 – 2 hours
When solid, pull the parchment paper out of the pan, put the block of fudge on a flat surface and cut into small squares
Enjoy! This will melt rather quickly — but it won't last long!

54. Choco – Almond Delights

Ingredients:
1 c. toasted hazelnuts
1 c. raw almonds
2/3 c. raw almond butter
5 Tbs. raw cacao powder (or unsweetened cocoa powder)
1/2 tsp. vanilla extract
1/4 c. unsweetened, shredded coconut
Stevia to taste

Instructions:
Combine all the ingredients, except for the coconut, in the food processor. Whir until smooth. This will take a few minutes and may require scraping down the sides of the bowl one or more times.

Line a mini muffin tin with plastic wrap. Spoon dollops of the sweet mixture into the lined tin cups and form into "mounds." Freeze until well formed. Remove mounds from plastic and tin and flip for presentation. Sprinkle with shredded coconut.

55. Peachy Creamy Peaches

Ingredients:
3 medium ripe peaches, cut in half with pit removed
1 tsp vanilla
1 can coconut milk, refrigerated
1/4 cup chopped walnuts
Cinnamon and stevia (to taste)

Instructions:
Place peaches on the grill with the cut side down first. Grill on medium-low heat until soft, about 3-5 minutes on each side.
Scoop cream off the top of the can of chilled coconut milk. Whip together coconut cream and vanilla with handheld mixer. Drizzle over each peach. Top with cinnamon and chopped walnuts to garnish.

56. Lemon-Coconut Petit Fours

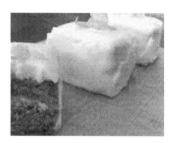

Ingredients:
For the Cake
1/2 cup coconut flour
1/2 cup coconut milk
3 eggs, separated
1/2 tsp vanilla
1/2 tsp baking soda
1/4 tsp low sodium salt
1 tsp lemon rind

Frosting
2/3 cup coconut cream (from the top of a can of coconut milk)
2 tbsp almond milk
1 tbsp Stevia
3 tsp lemon juice
¼ cup coconut oil, room temperature

Instructions
Separate the eggs with yolks in one bowl and whites in one large stainless steel, glass or ceramic bowl. When you go to whip the egg whites, it helps if they are at room temperature.
Combine coconut flour, milk, egg yolks, vanilla, baking soda, salt and lemon rind and mix.
Whip the egg whites until foamy and stiff peaks form. This is much easier if you have a stand mixer with the whisk attachment or a hand mixer. It is possible to do it by hand, but takes time.
Gently fold egg whites into the batter. Grease a standard sized loaf pan. Put batter in pan and even out the top with a spatula or spoon.
Bake in a 350° oven for 20-30 minutes or when a toothpick inserted comes out clean.

For the frosting

Coconut cream can be purchased in cans or you can skim the cream of the top of cans of coconut milk, however you may have to use multiple cans of coconut milk. Put coconut cream in a bowl and whisk for a few minutes to make it lighter and creamier.

Add coconut oil, milk, stevia and lemon juice and whisk until fully incorporated.

Allow the cake to cool completely before frosting. Once the cake has cooled, cut small squares or circles out of the cake and skim some cake off of the top with a knife to make it even. There will be leftover scraps, but they make a great snack!

Cut the squares in half and frost the middle. You can use the prepared frosting, but it will be very thin.

Drizzle the prepared frosting over the small cake squares and use a spatula or knife to frost the sides evenly. Once you've frosted each petit fours, refrigerate to allow the frosting to harden. Top with a bit of lemon rind.

Holiday Snacks

57. Holiday Breakfast Bonanza Muffins

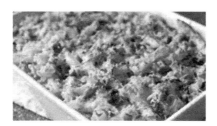

Ingredients:
8 eggs
1 cup diced broccoli
1 cup diced onion
1 cup diced mushrooms
low sodium salt and pepper, to taste
This recipe makes 8 muffins.

Instructions:
Preheat oven to 350 degrees F.
Dice all vegetables. You can add more or less of any of them, but keep the overall portion of vegetables the same for best results.
In a large mixing bowl, whisk together eggs, vegetables, low sodium salt, and pepper.
Pour mixture into a greased muffin pan, the mixture should evenly fill 8 muffin cups.
Bake 18-20 minutes, or until a toothpick inserted in the middle comes out clean.
Serve and enjoy! Leftovers can be saved in the refrigerator throughout the week.

58. Perfect Pumpkin Seeds

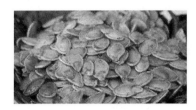

Ingredients:
1 cup of pumpkin (only seeds)
2 teaspoons of olive oil
1 tablespoon of chili powder (you may adjust it as per the taste you like)
1 teaspoon low sodium salt

Instructions:
Heat the pan (medium high heat) and place the pumpkin seeds.
After 3 to 5 minutes, you will hear the seeds making a crackling noise (some will even pop). You need to stir frequently.
Remove the pan and mix the seeds in olive oil, then low sodium salt and chili powder. Let it cool and then serve.

59. Gorgeous Spicy Nuts

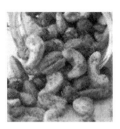

Ingredients:
2/3 cup of each (almonds, pecans and walnuts)
1 teaspoon of chili powder
½ teaspoon of cumin
½ teaspoon of black
pepper (ground)
½ teaspoon low sodium salt
1 tables

Instructions:
Heat the pan on medium heat and place the nuts and toast them until lightly browned.
Prepare the spice mixture, while the nuts are toasting.
Mix cumin, chili, low sodium salt and black pepper in a bowl and add the nuts (after coating it with olive oil).

60. Krunchy Yummy Kale Chips

Ingredients:
1 bunch of kale, washed and dried
2 tbsp olive oil
low sodium salt to taste

Instructions:
Preheat oven to 300 degrees. Remove the center stems and either tear or cut up the leaves.
Toss the kale and olive oil together in a large bowl; sprinkle with low sodium salt. Spread on a baking sheet
Bake at 300 degrees for 15 minutes or until crisp.

61. Divine Butternut Chips

Ingredients:
1 medium butternut squash (400g / 14.1 oz)
2 tbsp extra virgin coconut oil
1 tsp gingerbread spice mix (~ ½ tsp cinnamon, pinch nutmeg, ginger, cloves and allspice)
pinch low sodium salt (or more in case you don't use stevia and prefer the chips salty)

optional: 3-6 drops liquid Stevia extract

Instructions:
Preheat the oven to 125 C / 250 F. Peel the butternut squash and slice thinly on a mandolin. If you are using a knife, make sure the slices are no more than 1/8 inch (1/4 cm) thin. Place in a bowl.
In a small bowl, mix melted coconut oil, gingerbread spice mix and stevia.
Pour the oil mixture over the butternut squash and mix well to allow it everywhere.
Arrange the slices close to each other on a baking tray lined with parchment paper or a rack or an oven chip tray (you will need at least 2 of them).
Place in the oven and cook for about 1.5 hour or until crispy (the exact time depends on how thick the chips are).

62. Outstanding Orange Snack

Ingredients:
1 T. vanilla extract
½ t. natural orange flavor
Pinch low sodium salt
1 ½ t. liquid stevia to taste
8 T. vegetarian gelatin
1 can coconut milk
1 ½ C. water

Instructions:
Heat water and coconut milk over low heat until simmering.
Continue on low heat, slowly adding in each tablespoon of gelatin, whisking the entire time.
Add remaining ingredients and whisk until any clumps of gelatin are gone.
Pour into molds, and pour remaining liquid into 8X8 glass pan.
Put in fridge until solid. ...should pop out easily once hardened.

63. Pumpkin Vanilla Delight

Ingredients:
115g (1/2 cup) pumpkin seeds
1 tsp vanilla extract
2 tsp liquid stevia
Water (boiled)

Instructions:
Preheat oven to 150c.

In a medium bowl, combine the liquid stevia, and vanilla. Stir together to create a thick paste then add a small drop of boiled water to thin it out and create a runny syrup.

Pour in the pumpkin seeds and stir them around in the mixture to evenly coat them.

Dollop a generous tsp full of the pumpkin seeds onto a baking sheet, repeat until it's all used up and cook for 15-20 minutes until most of the seeds have browned (but don't let them burn!)

Take out of the oven and leave to cool for a few minutes. Once they've cooled a little (but are still warm) you can press the clusters together to make sure they don't fall apart. They will dry quickly.

Once they're cooled and dried, they're ready to eat! Enjoy on their own or served on top of your cereal.

64. Delectable Parsnip Chips

Ingredients:
500g (1.1 pounds) Parsnips
1/4 Cup Coconut Oil, Melted
3 Tablespoons liquid stevia

Instructions:
Preheat the oven to 200°C (392°F) and get out an oven proof dish.
Peel the parsnips and cut them into chip sized pieces and place into the oven proof dish.
Pour over the coconut oil and distribute evenly.
Drizzle over the liquid stevia and stir to combine well.
Place in the oven and cook for 15 minutes.
Remove from the oven and toss the parsnips over to allow the other side to brown.
Place back in the oven and cook for a further 10 to 15 minutes or until golden.

65. Anti-Aging Fruit Delights

Ingredients:
1 1/4 – 1/2 cups of pureed strawberries and raspberries
*If you prefer a less concentrated version, use 1 1/4 c fruit puree, and 1/4 c water!
4 – 5 tbsp vegetarian gelatin

Instructions:
Pureé the strawberries and raspberries.
In a small pan or pot on medium heat, whisk the gelatin into the fruit pureé until the gelatin is fully dissolved.
Pour the mixture into a glass pan. The smaller the size, the thicker the fruit snacks.
Chill the mixture for about 30 – 45 minutes in the fridge.
Cut into pieces and enjoy! Store in the fridge.

66. Power Snack

Ingredients:
1/2 Avocado
1/2 tsp Paprika
1/2 tsp low sodium salt
1/2 tsp Garlic Powder

Instructions:
Sprinkle with all the seasonings and enjoy.

67. Delish Cashew Butter Treats

Ingredients:
1 Cup Cashews
Half cup coconut flour
0.5 Cup Cashew Butter

Instructions:
Add the cashews and cashew butter and process until the mixture forms a dough ball.
Add coconut flour to harden the mixture. You may need to scrape down the sides and help the mixture along to form a dough ball.
Once a dough ball has formed, move the dough to a plate to ensure there are no accidents with the food processor blade.
Form the mixture into 16 equal sized balls, refrigerate for at least an hour to harden and enjoy!

Holiday Smoothie Delight

68. Gorgeous Berry Smoothie

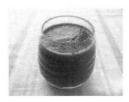

Ingredients:
½ cup frozen blueberries or 1 cup fresh blueberries
15 oz coconut milk
Stevia to taste
1 scoop of hemp protein
¼ teaspoon cinnamon (optional)

Instructions:
Place all ingredients into a blender.
Blend until mixed thoroughly.
Serve right away.

69. Tempting Coconut Berry Smoothie

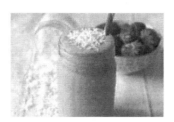

Ingredients:
½ Cup Frozen Blackberries
½ Frozen Banana
1 Teaspoon Chia Seeds
¼ Inch Piece of Fresh Ginger
½ Cup Almond
Coconut Milk
1 scoop of HEMP protein
2 Tablespoons Toasted Coconut

Instructions:
Combine all the ingredients in a blender and process until smooth.

70. Volumptious Vanilla Hot Drink

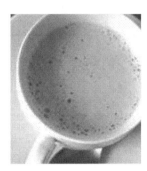

Ingredients:
3 cups unsweetened almond milk (or 1 1/2 cup full fat coconut milk + 1 1/2 cups water)
Stevia to taste
1 scoop of hemp protein
1/2 Tbsp. ground cinnamon (or more to taste)
1/2 Tbsp. vanilla extract

Instructions:
Place the almond milk into a pitcher. Place ground cinnamon, hemp, vanilla extract in a small saucepan over medium high heat. Heat until the pure liquid stevia is just melted and then pour the pure liquid stevia mixture into the pitcher. Stir until the pure liquid stevia is well combined with the almond milk. Place the pitcher in the fridge and allow to chill for at least two hours. Stir well before serving.

71. Almond Butter Smoothies

Ingredients:
1 scoop of hemp protein
1 Tablespoon natural almond butter
1 cup of hemp milk
1 banana, preferably frozen for a creamier shake
few ice cubes

Instructions:
Blend all ingredients together and enjoy!

72. Choco Walnut Delight

Ingredients:
1 scoop Hemp Protein
30g dark sugar free chocolate broken up.
50g walnuts chopped/crushed (depending on desired texture)
250ml hemp milk or nut milk alternative
Handful of ice cubes, the more you use the thicker it will be.

Instructions:
Blend everything together in a strong blender until thoroughly processed, and enjoy!
Makes 2, and can be stored in the fridge overnight.

73. Raspberry Hemp Smoothie

Ingredients:
1 cup hemp milk or milk alternative
1/2 cup raspberries (fresh or frozen)
2 tablespoons hemp protein powder
Stevia to taste
3 to 4 ice cubes

Instructions:
Add ingredients to a blender and blend until smooth.

74. Choco Banana Smoothie

Ingredients:
1 cup milk or milk alternative
2 peeled frozen bananas
4 ice cubes
2 tablespoons hulled hemp seed
2 tablespoons hemp protein powder
1 tablespoons organic cocoa powder
5-7 drops liquid stevia to sweeten
1/4 teaspoon cinnamon
1/4 teaspoon vanilla

Instructions:
Put all ingredients into blender. Blend until smooth.

75. Blueberry Almond Smoothie

Ingredients:
1 c almond milk
1 c frozen unsweetened blueberries
1 Tbsp cold-pressed organic flaxseed oil
2 tblsp hemp protein powder

Instructions:
Combine milk and blueberries in blender, and blend for 1 minute.
Transfer to glass, and stir in flaxseed oil.

76. Hazelnut Butter and Banana Smoothie

Ingredients:
½ c nut milk
½ c hemp milk
2 Tbsp creamy natural unsalted hazelnut butter
¼ very ripe banana
stevia drops to taste
4 ice cubes
2 tblsp hemp protein powder

Instructions:
Combine ingredients in a blender. Process until smooth.
Pour into a tall glass and serve.

77. Vanilla Blueberry Smoothie

Ingredients:
2 cups hemp milk
1 c fresh blueberries
Handful of ice OR 1 cup frozen blueberries
1 Tbsp flaxseed oil
2 tblsp hemp protein powder

Instructions:
Combine milk, and fresh blueberries plus ice (or frozen blueberries) in a blender.
Blend for 1 minute, transfer to a glass, and stir in flaxseed oil.

78. Chocolate Raspberry Smoothie

Ingredients:
1 cup almond milk
¼ c chocolate chips-sugar free
1 c fresh raspberries
2 tsp hemp protein powder
Handful of ice OR 1 cup frozen raspberries

Instructions:
COMBINE ingredients in a blender.
Blend for 1 minute, transfer to a glass, and eat with a spoon.

79. Peach Smoothie

Ingredients:
1 cup hemp milk
1 c frozen unsweetened peaches
2 tsp cold-pressed organic flaxseed oil (MUFA)
2 tsp hemp protein powder

Instructions:
PLACE milk and frozen, unsweetened peaches in blender and blend for 1 minute.
Transfer to glass, and stir in flaxseed oil.

80. Zesty Citrus Smoothie

Ingredients:
1 cup almond milk
half cup lemon juice
1 med orange peeled, cleaned, and sliced into sections
Handful of ice
1 Tbsp flaxseed oil
2 tsp hemp protein powder

Instructions:
COMBINE milk, lemon juice, orange, and ice in a blender.
Blend for 1 minute, transfer to a glass, and stir in flaxseed oil.

81. Apple Smoothie

Ingredients:
½ cup hemp milk
1 cup hemp milk
1 tsp apple pie spice
1 med apple peeled and chopped
2 Tbsp cashew butter
Handful of ice
2 tblsp hemp protein powder

Instructions:
COMBINE ingredients in a blender.
Blend for 1 minute, transfer to a glass, and eat with a spoon.

82. Pineapple Smoothie

Ingredients:
1 cup almond milk
4 oz fresh pineapple
Handful of ice
2 tblsp hemp protein powder
1 Tbsp cold-pressed organic flaxseed oil

Instructions:
PLACE milk, canned pineapple in blender, add of ice, and whip for 1 minute.
Transfer to glass and stir in flaxseed oil.

83. Strawberry Smoothie

Ingredients:
1 cup almond milk
1 c frozen, unsweetened strawberries
2 tblsp hemp protein powder
2 tsp cold-pressed organic flaxseed oil

Instructions:
COMBINE milk and strawberries in blender.
Blend, transfer to glass, and stir in flaxseed oil.

84. Pineapple Coconut Deluxe Smoothie

Ingredients:
1 C pineapple chunks
1 C coconut milk
1/2 C pineapple juice
1 ripe banana
1/2 – 3/4 C ice cubes
Pure liquid stevia to taste
1 tablespoon hemp protein powder

Instructions:
In a blender, combine the pineapple chunks, coconut milk, banana, ice and pure liquid stevia.
Puree until smooth.
Pour into 2 large glasses.
Garnish with a pineapple wedge if desired.

85. Divine Vanilla Smoothie

Ingredients:
1 cup coconut or almond milk
¼ cup almond butter
1 tsp vanilla paste, (or vanilla extract)
2 cups ice
Vanilla liquid, seeds or powder, to taste
Vanilla or plain hemp Protein Powder – 1 tablespoon

Instructions:
Add all ingredients except ice to blender. Puree well.
Add ice and blend until ice is all crushed and smoothie is well blended and smooth.
Pour into two glasses and serve immediately.

NOTES
Add more or less ice to make the smoothie thinner or thicker consistency.
Great for a post workout smoothie!

86. Coco Orange Delish Smoothie

Ingredients:
1/2 cup fresh squeezed orange juice (I used 1 1/2 oranges)
1 tablespoon hemp protein powder
1/2 cup full fat coconut milk from the can (not the box!)
1 teaspoon vanilla
1/2 -1 cup crushed ice

Instructions:
Add all ingredients to a blender.
Blend until smooth and add ice as needed to get the consistency you like.

87. Baby Kale Pineapple Smoothie

Ingredients:
1 cup almond milk
1/2 cup frozen pineapple
1 cup Kale
1 tablespoon hemp protein powder

Instructions:
Place the almond milk, pineapple, and greens in the blender and blend until smooth.

88. Sumptuous Strawberry Coconut Smoothie

Ingredients:
1 cup coconut milk
1 frozen banana, sliced
2 cups frozen strawberries
1 teaspoon vanilla extract
1 tablespoon hemp protein powder

Instructions:
Add all ingredients to blender and blend until smooth.

89. Blueberry Bonanza Smoothies

Ingredients:
1/4 cup canned coconut or almond milk
1/2 cup water
1 medium banana, sliced
1 cup frozen blueberries
1 tablespoon raw almonds

Instructions:
Add coconut milk, water, banana, blueberries and almonds to blender container.
Cover and blend until smooth. Pour into 2 glasses.

90. Divine Peach Coconut Smoothie

Ingredients:
1 cup full fat coconut milk, chilled
1 cup ice
2 large fresh peaches, peeled and cut into chunks
Fresh lemon zest, to taste
1 tablespoon hemp protein powder

Instructions:
Add coconut milk, ice and peaches blender. Using a zester, add a few gratings of fresh lemon zest. Blend on high speed until smooth.

91. Tantalizing Key Lime Pie Smoothie

Ingredients:
1 cup coconut milk
1 cup ice
1/2 avocado
zest and juice of 2 limes
Pure liquid stevia to taste
1 tablespoon hemp protein powder

Instructions:
Add all ingredients to Vitamix or blender and blend until smooth.

92. High Protein and Nutritional Delish Smoothie

Ingredients:
1 cup almond milk
1/2 Avocado
4 Strawberries
1/2 Bananas (Very ripe)
1/2 cup Raw Kale or spinach
1/4 cup Carrot Juice) water can be used
1 cup Coconut Yogurt..or almond milk)
1 tablespoon hemp protein powder

Instructions:
Add everything to your blender, and blend to your preferred consistency
More water or ice can be added to help with your preferred texture/thickness.

93. Pineapple Protein Smoothie

Ingredients:
1 cup (135g) pineapple chunks
1 cup (200g) coconut milk (fresh or tinned)
½ med (65g) banana
¼ cup (65g) ice cubes
¼ tsp vanilla bean powder
pinch low sodium salt
1 tablespoon hemp protein powder

Instructions:
Peel pineapple and chop into small chunks.
Put everything into a high speed blender and blend until smooth.

94. Raspberry Coconut Smoothie

Ingredients:
½ - 1 cup coconut milk (depending on how thick you like it)
1 medium banana, peeled sliced and frozen
2 teaspoons coconut extract (optional)
1 cup frozen raspberries
1 tablespoon hemp protein powder

optional: shredded coconut flakes, and stevia to taste

Instructions:
Add coconut milk, frozen banana slices and coconut extract to your blender.
Pulse 1-2 minutes until smooth.
Add frozen raspberries and continue to pulse until smooth.
Pour into your serving glass, top with a couple of raspberries and a little shredded coconut, and enjoy!

95. Ginger Carrot Protein Smoothie

Ingredients:
3/4 cup carrot juice
1 tablespoon hemp protein powder
1 tablespoon hulled hemp seeds
1/2 apple
3 to 4 ice cubes
1/2 inch piece fresh ginger

Instructions:
Add to a blender and blend until smooth.

The Paleo Ketogenic Holiday Recipes for Beginners By Beran Parry

Holiday Sumptuous Soup

96. Wonderful Watercress Soup

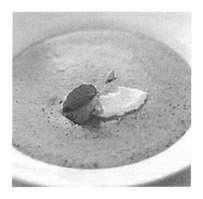

Ingredients:
1 quart low sodium chicken stock
1 medium leek
1 bunch water cress
1 large onion
1/2 celeriac root skinned and chopped
2 cups diced chicken breast – organic
low sodium salt and pepper to taste

Instructions:
Gently heat the chicken stock in the pot.
In the fry pan sauté the onion, leek and celeriac until soft.
Place the onion, leek, chicken and celeriac in the pot of stock reserving 1/3 aside.
Season with low sodium salt and pepper.
Add the bunch of watercress and simmer a few minutes until it is wilted.
With the immersion blender blend the soup.
Add the chopped vegetables that you reserved, back into the pot.

97. Celery Cashew Cream Soup

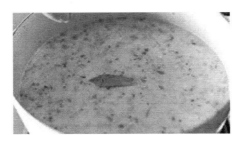

Ingredients:
300 grams celery, washed and chopped
1 small onion, chopped
1.5 tbsp olive oil
500 mls vegetable stock
40 grams cashew nuts
low sodium salt and pepper to taste

Instructions:
Heat the olive oil in a large saucepan then add the celery and onion, stir to coat with oil. Turn the heat low and put the lid on leaving the vegetables to sweat for 5 minutes.
Add the garlic, give a quick stir then add the vegetable stock and simmer for 10 minutes.
Add the cashew nuts to the saucepan and simmer for another 5 minutes or until the celery is cooked through.
Tip the soup mix into a blender and purée until smooth.
Season with the low sodium salt and pepper and serve.

98. Tempting Tomato Basil Soup

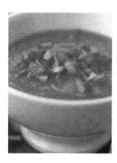

Ingredients:
4 cans whole tomatoes, crushed Note: check for ones without added sugar or salt!
4 cups tomato juice and part low sodium vegetable broth or chicken broth (I use 2 cups tomato juice and 2 cups low sodium chicken broth)
12 or 14 fresh basil leaves
1 cup coconut milk
Low sodium salt and cracked black pepper to taste

Instructions:
Combine tomatoes, juice and/or broth in stockpot. Simmer 30 minutes.
Purée, along with basil leaves, in small batches in a food processor, blender or better yet, a hand-held immersion blender right in the pot.
Return to pot and add coconut milk while stirring over low heat.

99. Delicious Lemon-Garlic Soup

Option – add 6 shrimps

Ingredients:
1 tablespoon olive oil
1 tablespoon crushed and chopped fresh garlic
6 cups good-quality low sodium shellfish stock (or mushroom or chicken stock)
2 eggs
1/3 to 1/2 cup fresh lemon juice
1 tablespoon coconut flour for thickening
1/4 teaspoon ground white pepper
chopped fresh cilantro or parsley, if desired

Instructions:
In a 4-quart pot, heat the olive oil over medium-high heat and saute the garlic for 1-2 minutes, or until just fragrant. Do not let the garlic brown.
Reserve 1/2 cup of the stock to mix with the eggs. Pour the remaining 5 1/2 cups of stock into the pot with the garlic. Let the mixture come to a simmer.
In a small bowl, whisk together the eggs, lemon juice, arrowroot, white pepper, and half of a cup of reserved stock. Pour the mixture into the simmering stock and stir until it all thickens--this will only take a few minutes.
Serve the soup hot, sprinkled with fresh cilantro or parsley.

100. Turkey Squash Soup

Ingredients:
1 large acorn squash
1/2 teaspoon olive oil
low sodium salt and pepper to taste
2 cups chicken or vegetable stock
1/4 cup coconut milk
1-2 turkey breasts shredded
3/4 teaspoon ground ginger
1 tablespoon coconut aminos
Pinch or two of cayenne pepper
Pomegranate seeds and/or sliced almonds, for serving

Instructions:
Preheat the oven to 400. Cut the acorn squash in half and scoop out the seeds and pulp. Brush each half with about 1/4 teaspoon olive oil and sprinkle with low sodium salt and pepper. Place in a foil-lined baking pan and roast, cut sides up, until fork tender (about an hour).
When the squash is cool enough to handle, scoop out the flesh and place it in a medium saucepan, or in a blender if you don't have an immersion blender. Add the remaining ingredients and process with an immersion blender (or regular blender) until smooth. Place the saucepan over medium heat and cook, stirring often, until heated through. Serve hot or warm, with pomegranate seeds and/or sliced almonds.

Bibliography

Eating Disorders and the Brain by Bryan Lask

The Paleo Diet Revised: by Dr Loren Cordain PhD

The Protein Boost Diet by Dr Ridha Arem

Eating Well: How to build good eating habits to have your perfect body and overcome eating disorder

Stephen Ecker

The Anderson Method: The Secret to Permanent Weight Loss

William Anderson, Dr. Mark Lupo

The Vitamin D Solution: A 3-Step Strategy to Cure Our Most Common Health Problems

Michael F. Holick Ph.D. M.D., Andrew Weil

OBESITY GENES and their Epigenetic Modifiers

by James Baird

Genes and Obesity (Progress in Molecular Biology & Translational Science)

by C. Bouchard

Practical Manual of Clinical Obesity

by Robert Kushner and Victor Lawrence

The Epigenetics Revolution: How Modern Biology Is Rewriting Our Understanding of Genetics, Disease, and Inheritance...by Nessa Carey

Transgenerational Epigenetics by Trygve Tollefsbol

The Evolution of Obesity by Michael L. Power and Jay Schulkin

The China Study: by Thomas Campbell and T. Colin Campbell

Death by food pyramid by Denise Minger

Primal blueprint by Mark Sissons

The magnesium miracle Dr Carolyn Deane

What are you hungry for by deepak chopra

Gut and Psychology Syndrome: by Dr Natasha Campbell-McBride

BEFORE YOU GO

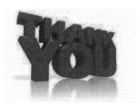

I am so delighted that you have chosen this book and it's been a pleasure writing it for you. My mission is to help as many readers as possible to benefit from the content you have just been reading. So many of us are able to take new information and apply it to our lives with really positive and long lasting consequences and it is my wish that you have been able to take value from the information I have presented.

Thank you for staying with me during this book and for reading it through to the end. I really hope that you have enjoyed the contents and that's why I appreciate your feedback so much. If you could take a couple of minutes to review the book, your views will help me to create more material that you find beneficial.

I am always delighted to hear from my readers and you can email me personally at beranparry@gmail.com if you have any questions about this book or future books. Let us know how we can help you by sending a message to the same email address.

Thanks again for your support and encouragement. I really look forward to reading your review.

Just go to the Amazon book product page to post your review

Stay Healthy!

The Paleo Ketogenic Holiday Recipes for Beginners By Beran Parry

Which of Your Wellbeing Challenges can I help You with?

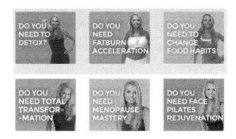

Please search this page over the internet
beranparry.com/courses/

FOR MORE FROM BERAN PARRY

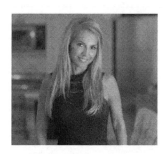

Please search this page over the internet
beranparry.com/

MORE FREE GIFTS

Take YOUR Free Toxin Test

Get my Free Face Pilates EBook

Join my Free EClub and Get my 3 Best Fat Loss Recipes

Get Your Free Belly Buster 101 Ways to Banish Your Belly Fat

The Paleo Ketogenic Holiday Recipes for Beginners By Beran Parry

As a special seasonal gift I would like to offer you my 5 day Paleo Detox at a 50% discount to do before or after the Holiday Season. It contains the following exciting elements

Delicious Recipes,

Stunning Detox Menu's,

Detoxifying Pilates Exercise Videos,

A Daily Detox Face Pilates Program,

Guided Detox Meditations,

FREE Bonus Recipe Books,

FREE Stress Release System

Here is more info and the coupon code

beranparry.com/midlife-fatburn-detox

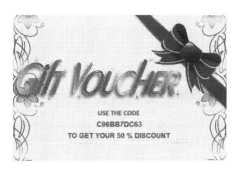

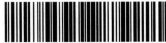

Made in the USA
Middletown, DE
19 November 2018